Autism Rewrote My Family

Sarah Vanis

NEW HAVEN PUBLISHING

Published 2022
First Edition
NEW HAVEN PUBLISHING LTD
www.newhavenpublishingltd.com
newhavenpublishing@gmail.com

All Rights Reserved
The rights of Sarah Vanis, as the author of this work, have been asserted in accordance with the Copyrights, Designs and Patents Act 1988.
No part of this book may be re-printed or reproduced or utilized in any form or by any electronic, mechanical or other means, now unknown or hereafter invented, including photocopying, and recording, or in any information storage or retrieval system, without the written permission of the
Author and Publisher.

Cover Design © Pete Cunliffe

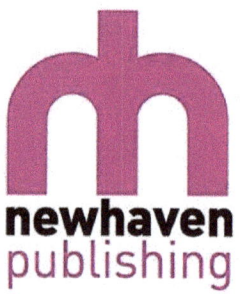

Copyright © 2022 Sarah Vanis
All rights reserved
ISBN: 978-1-949515-34-3

My heartfelt thanks go to the following people who helped us seek some light:

Teddie Dahlin, my publisher, who took a leap of faith in helping to share my writing to help others. I am eternally grateful.

My wonderful colleague, Dr Prathibha, for your open arms.

My therapists; without you all we would still be struggling.

My mother, who did her best in the way she knew how.

My children, for your unconditional love and care.

And my rock, baby I forever love you.

Foreword

I write this with love. Three years ago, I wrote a book about my experiences with anorexia nervosa, and about how I found hope and healing through yoga and Ayurveda. Little did I know then that the anorexia would reveal its ugly head again. This started a journey that took both me and my family by surprise. I discovered I had autism. I was predestined to the anorexia as an undiagnosed middle-aged woman.

Mental illness I know. Autism I did not. I struggled to understand what autism was, and it was profound. It also led to a diagnosis for my three children. Together my husband and I navigated what it meant to have four people in our family with a confirmed diagnosis. As I tried to find us support, I found the lack of services and the long waiting lists confusing. The terminology was all so new. It was almost like learning a new language.

I write this book now, examining my life through the lens of autism. Whilst previously I had a 'deficit' approach to life, as a client of the mental health system, now I find hope. I am not broken. I never was. My mental health was never a deficit, even though the system and my extended family may have instigated this response. I am a whole being, capable of living a happy and fulfilling life as a productive member of society - just a different kind of society member, which I am proud to be.

I write this book to suggest strategies and techniques which will hopefully help make the navigation of an intricate system a little more easy for those who are newly diagnosed or those who are seeking answers. If you are doubting getting a diagnosis, I say go for it. Don't wait. Find someone you like and book in with them. And if you don't feel they are right, do it again. I know it is costly; I know the experience is harrowing. The experience of a diagnosis changed my life, the lives of my children, and our whole family, and I hope it helps touch your heart as well.

Contents

Chapter 1 - The Moment the World as We Knew it Changed — 7

Chapter 2 - Rewriting the Story — 14

Chapter 3 - Diagnosis Runs In the Family — 16

Chapter 4 - Rewind. Re-evaluating to Find a New Identity – Primary School — 19

Chapter 5 - Rewind. Re-evaluating to Find a New Identity - High School — 25

Chapter 6 - Leaving School and Entering a Different Domain - Eating Disorder City Here I Come! — 29

Chapter 7 - Growing Up - Moving On — 33

Chapter 8 - What is Autism? — 37

Chapter 9 - Adult Late Diagnosis Autism — 41

Chapter 10 - Child Diagnosis — 51

Chapter 11 - Parenting with Autism - Recognising the Traits — 66

Chapter 12 - Strategies for Our Parenting — 71

Chapter 13 - Autism and Relationships — 77

Chapter 14 - Autism Burnout — 91

Chapter 15 - Living with Autism - Rewriting the Story — 107

Epilogue - New Year 2022 — 148

Appendix — 158

References — 161

Chapter 1
The Moment the World As We Knew It Changed

Press play. Repeat. Stop. Now process. Sometimes processing doesn't work anymore because there is no longer any energy left to make sense of it all. Try to press play. It's broken. Now there's trouble. This is what my life felt like for so long. I was a cassette tape getting stuck time and time again. And I didn't know how to break the pattern.

Three years ago, I tried to fit into society. I really did try and fit. In fact, I had been trying for 43 years, to be exact. I just couldn't seem to work out why I was on the outskirts, and I was doing my darned level best to fit in. Three years ago, I gave up. My play button was on stuck on pause and the cassette tape was wearing out.

I ended up contacting the mental health team at the hospital. Something had to give. I had failed in my quest to overcome mental illness and it was consuming me, so much so that I was having difficulties seeing my way out, and planning how to escape. I drove at times imagining what it would feel like to hit that tree on my left at full speed. I was eating the same thing day in and day out. I was starting to think that my eating disorder, which I had worked so hard to combat, was coming back, and with a vengeance. Quite frankly, I was in trouble and no one knew. I was the queen of masking, and running a successful full-time business. But the play button was broken.

I was accepted as an outpatient, and I was a friggin' mess. I had nothing left. The psych nurse asked me to explain what had happened. For a little bit, I took my finger off the pause button and began to share my story.

Growing up had been rough. The oldest of four, being the only female and a sensitive child had left me vulnerable to becoming the scapegoat for a couple of parents who were both pretty stuffed up. Both had traumatic histories and most of the time they were at each other's throats. Growing up, for me, was isolating.

I remember my mum used to say to me: you blame everyone for bad things and never take ownership. She would say that not everyone can be bad. I didn't really get it. I just never seemed to fit in. It didn't help that my father was pretty cruel. Things like 'go kill yourself' and 'you're so fat no one could love you 'were common phrases I grew up with. Needless to say, I was on the path to an eating disorder. And if there is one thing I am good at, it is commitment. I did my eating disorder proud! I was hospitalised many times, and consequently in my teens and early 20s I was too sick to do much at all. I never did get that love from my father in the end, and I haven't seen him for over 20 years now.

Despite all this baggage, I married a terrific bloke. Somehow, he managed to weave his way into my heart and I grew out of anorexia and addiction and really wanted to become someone better. I had hope for the first time. We married. My siblings and his sister appeared to get on well. Fast forward 10 years, they were getting on a little too well. I started hearing stories of how they were all holidaying together. Hmm. I was feeling left out. I was feeling my children were being left out from sharing with their cousins. What was happening?

My husband and I decided to split the intervention. He would deal with his family and I would deal with my family. I did what I do best. I spoke to my siblings. I used my very best voice to de-emotionalise and only talk with the facts. This was to make sure I didn't get upset and to help me communicate clearly. It backfired. I was accused of being unreasonable and cold.

My husband let the whole situation go. He wasn't as upset as me and didn't approach the issue with his family. This went on for another two years. I would try and talk, to my mum as well. Every family gathering was filled with anxiety and I would need to debrief with my husband for hours afterwards, constantly analysing every sentence and every action. We hardly saw the family anymore. No one ever visited us. I felt lonely and trashy. What was I doing wrong? I just couldn't seem to work it out.

My husband and I took some time out and went to Bali for ten days. We left our three kids with his parents at our home. It was a rarity for them to visit us in the country. My husband became sick, and for five days he was so unwell I called the hospital whilst we were in Bali. He was severely dehydrated. We called home to speak to the kids and I could see my sister-in-law's kid in the background. Oh no. My sister-in-law was at our place - over two and a half hours away, with her kids sleeping in my bed to boot. My brother and mother were there as well.

This was the last straw. It was too much for me to process. Press play. Repeat. Process. The processing had stopped. I was stuck on pause in my cassette tape. I got the message: I was crap. It was all my fault. My family would be happier and more connected if I wasn't there. I had my evidence, didn't I?

My husband and I came home both wiped out. I tried to talk and use my very best factual voice to tell my extended family how I felt. Inside I felt like I was dying. It was too much to bear anymore. My eating became restricted. I started losing interest in business. I was just feeling like crap. My husband and I spoke constantly about family and I was trying so hard to work it all out so I could make it better. I was getting messages from both sides of the family that I was causing trouble. These messages are unrepeatable and really damming to me. I just didn't know why I was so awful. At the same time, I was trying to keep up a façade that all was well to those around me. The double life was exhausting. How could I be successful when those who were supposed to love me didn't want to be around me?

Christmas was painful. No one wanted to spend Christmas with us. We saw the in-laws the next day and were given the leftovers from their Christmas dinner, which they had enjoyed with my sister-in-law and her husband's family. They arrived with presents from the sister-in-law for our kids. Huge, expensive presents. I didn't understand. Maybe if I just went and disappeared, their lives would all be better? I didn't cope.

I yelled at my husband to try and make sense of all of this. My husband blew up. He put the presents in the bin; the kids screamed; the leftover dinner went in the bin. I screamed. I was lost and alone. This was it. Play was broken and repeat was stuck. Pause wasn't even in the picture any more. I had the cassette tapes telling me the same messages over and over and over.

So the hospital was my salvation. I had to find a way out of this crap, to make it better for my family. At the first session I was told to go on antipsychotics immediately. Oh, come on. For years I had worked my way out of an eating disorder and all the medication crap to become an advocate for yoga and Ayurveda, and now I was being told to take some pretty serious medication. I was so distraught that I agreed. This resulted in my thinking becoming foggy. I couldn't find my words: I could see them in my head but I couldn't hold onto them. But I didn't care. The side effects of the antipsychotics were a huge break. I just didn't care.

I was told I would be treated for a relapse of the eating disorder. I was weighed. I am always weighed backwards. I sat with the mandatory dietician. What a joke. I was pre-diagnosed by the psych nurse. She told me I also had borderline personality disorder and it would be confirmed the next week by the psychiatrist.

What the hell? There was something else wrong with me, on top of the eating disorder? I felt like a bad person. I lived for that appointment with the psychiatrist. I needed this new diagnosis of borderline personality disorder to be confirmed. In the meantime, I researched borderline personality disorder like crazy. I needed to know all I could to beat these disorders and to not affect my children. I felt like I was fighting for my life, hidden from sight of the public, whilst also maintaining a business.

The psychiatrist appointment came, and it was a friggin' joke. This big fat middle aged man sat back in his chair and asked what I wanted. I said a diagnosis. He said: what do you think? I said, what do you mean? You are the expert? The psych nurse sat in the corner and watched me. I felt like a frightened rabbit, cornered in a hole. I couldn't escape. I had obeyed their rules; I was taking their medication. I was lost. He was supposed to tell me. I panicked and became hysterical.

Later I called the psych nurse and said I was upset. It was Friday at 4pm. She told me to keep on the medications and wait until she saw me next week. I felt abused and tormented. I stayed on the medication.

Things continued to go downhill from there. This psych nurse was meant to be the best for treating eating disorders, but she told me I now had borderline personality disorder, and she wasn't allowed to see me more than once a week, and only for a limited time. I would be referred on. Press play. Repeat. The cassette was different though, so different from the two sessions a week we had agreed on. I once again had proof: I was worthless.

I contacted my brothers and sisters-in-law. I also contacted my mother. I did this through email, sending links to easy-to-understand YouTube videos explaining borderline personality disorder. My research had shown that borderline personality disorder has a strong genetic component. I wanted to reach out and tell them I was sorry. That I didn't mean any fighting. Perhaps, if they knew about my diagnosis, they could be on the lookout for symptoms in their own family, which would prevent any one of their children going through my pain. The response? Nothing. Press Play. Repeat. Dumb cassette tape.

I may think I am worthless, but I am a fighter. I have to be to have made it this far, out of a debilitating eating disorder, overcoming a drug addiction and fighting alcoholism. Ok. Back to the drawing board.

I had heard borderline personality disorder was best cured by a treatment called dialectical behavioural therapy (DBT). There was a place in Richmond that was the best. It was a government run service and I didn't have health insurance. I was on the wait list. The twelve month wait list.

In the meantime, though, I found a local service where I lived. Oh my gosh! The planets were now starting to line up and I could beat this borderline personality disorder. I had found hope.

Sometimes you meet a therapist and you get a feeling. I had been around long enough now, and I should have listened. It didn't feel right. The DBT group was put online as a result of Covid-19, which was fair enough. I was late for the first session; I was gutted, so I jumped online, already panicked. The therapist just kept on talking, not acknowledging I had come on. Ok. Words were flying in the chat box and I was trying to follow the conversation. At one point I tipped over the edge and I was triggered by another group member's personal disclosure. No one knew I was triggered. Half the cameras were turned off and I was having trouble analysing everyone. And those bloody chat boxes. I asked if the chats could stop. All hell broke loose. To cut a long story short, I was told no, and it became personal amongst the group members. My panic went to distress.

Afterwards, my husband saw my face. I was debriefed with the co-facilitator, who agreed the chat was distracting and the disclosure may have been a trigger. I continued with the program, and sat with the therapist for individual sessions, but I could not understand the program. I was trying to make sense of it all and the DBT process. When was I to use the distress phone call? I felt distress up to ten times a day. Please explain it to me. For some reason, she couldn't. I felt we were butting heads.

I enrolled in the next module. Again, during individual sessions, I tried to make sense of the program, but I was becoming guarded. Only a handful of group members participated in the sessions and many cameras were turned off. One particular group member continued to disclose personal information and I felt unsafe. I told the therapist I felt sorry for her during the sessions because she answered all her own questions. She told me her team of therapists had decided in a group meeting eight weeks ago that I wasn't suitable for the program and they all wanted me out. She told me she had fought for me to stay in. Press Play. Repeat. Stuck on repeat. Again, I had evidence that I was hopeless. I wasn't even good enough for the one therapy that was supposed to cure me, or at least help me to manage borderline personality disorder. Where was I to go now? That tree and my car were looking mighty good again.

Persistence might be my middle name. I have a book with every therapist in our local area, and I started ringing around. I took notes. I researched as much as I could about the ones that sounded ok. One therapist said she didn't treat eating disorders, but as I was hanging up, she asked me to tell her a little bit more. I went with my gut. I made an appointment to see her.

She became a confidante. I trusted her. She read my book on anorexia. She researched. She listened. She asked me to change medications. I could think a little more now. In time, I would stop all medications. As we spoke, she watched me transition between extremely suicidal to downright depressed. The swings were hard to deal with for me, let alone for the rest of my family. I was still managing to keep up the mask of a business owner, but I was becoming fatigued. One day she said to me: Stop. I pressed Stop. She asked me to get assessed by a prominent therapist in women's mental health.

The result was that I was diagnosed with complex post traumatic stress disorder (CPTSD) and premenstrual dysphoric disorder (PMDD). CPTSD is a complicated way of saying that repeated traumas have caused stress; PTSD is generally considered to relate to one traumatic event. This I would agree with. I had CPTSD. The PMDD is likened to a period on steroids: mood swings out of this world, suicide ideations and aggression to the extremes.

I went home and researched. I bought books on CPTSD and PMDD. I joined Facebook groups. I listed to podcasts. I was put on the pill. Say goodbye to any libido. It didn't work. I was put on anti-depressants. I felt worse than ever. I was diagnosed with attention deficient disorder (ADD) by another psychiatrist, and put on another medication. I was still sliding downhill.

My therapist told me I should feel relief after a month of ADD medication. I didn't. The psychiatrist wanted to increase the dose to four times as much. STOP. My turn to stop. No more medication. I couldn't get my words out, even though no one around me was noticing; my husband and therapist were the only ones who knew how bad things were becoming.

At our next session, my therapist looked at me. We went through all the therapies we had tried: cognitive behavioural therapy, schema-based therapy, dialectical behavioural therapy, antipsychotics, antidepressants, anti-ADD medication, the pill. Nothing was working. She told me it was time for me to be tested for autism, and I just looked at her. Seriously?

Press Play. Stop. Rewind. I put in a new cassette tape. This was the cassette tape that was correct. It was about to rerecord my whole life and rewrite my story. I was diagnosed with autism level 2 at age 43 years.

Chapter 2
Rewriting the Story

I had a disability. My therapist rejigged every concept I ever had of myself. She said I suffered terribly from anxiety. No… I had always thought of this as aggression. She said my anxiety manifested as aggression. What? I had to rethink everything.

I went home and researched. I bought books on female autism. I bought books on adult female autism. I joined Facebook groups on autism for females. I listened to podcasts on female adult autism. I had autism. It fitted. I had a disability.

Again, I contacted my brothers and sisters-in-law. Again, I contacted my mother. Again, I did this through email, with links to easy-to-understand YouTube videos on autism spectrum disorder. My research had shown that autism also has a strong genetic component, stronger than borderline personality disorder. I really wanted to reach out to them and tell them I was sorry, that I didn't mean any fighting, and that it might have been my fixation and lack of social comprehension that made things difficult for us. Again, I thought if they knew, they could be on the lookout for symptoms in their own family. This would prevent any one of their children going through my pain, and early diagnosis means early intervention. The response? A really aggressive message from my brother, which I would never share in public, denying any possibility of me having autism and damning all my family. My brother is a nurse and his response shocked me. Press play. Stop. Remove that cassette tape. It is now dangerous to have contact from my siblings.

I met with my mother face to face. I showed her, for the first time in all of my history of hospitalisation and health professional support, all my assessment reports, and allowed her to read them. I showed her the message from my brother. Initially she demonstrated support. A few weeks later, though, I received a letter from her in which she denied my diagnosis, instead blaming my past drug use and anorexia for my current position. She also decided my misfortune was a result of a bump on the head I experienced when I was six years old. I was to blame for the family dysfunction; and I had ruined Christmas. I chose to no longer press play. My mother's disbelief hurt. There cannot be any more repeats or any more pauses. The stop button is now jammed on. This cassette tape is also removed. Now I grow.

Chapter 3
Diagnosis Runs In The Family

We have three children. During my research into autism I started recognising traits of autism level 2 in my daughter. Oh my gosh. What had I done? Please no, don't tell me she has autism. The buck was meant to stop with me. I had to know. True to autism, I became fixated. I researched questionnaires and had her complete them. I was aware I was not trained; however, I had been informally training for this my whole life.

My son wanted to do the questionnaires too. Oh, goodness, no. His results were showing high levels of social anxiety. Now, I am not a psychologist, but I am a great researcher. I scoured through diagnosis books and presented a case to my husband. At first, he was in denial.

I talked to my therapist. We talked about Munchausen's syndrome. I had to think. Surely I wasn't making this up? Again, I presented a case to my husband about my daughter. I was also starting to think my youngest daughter, my baby, also had traits of autism. This was becoming a bit too much for my husband: a year ago, he had a wife with a re-occurring eating disorder, then his wife was also diagnosed with an untreatable but manageable mental health illness of borderline personality disorder… now suddenly she has a disability? And is now saying his three children also have a disability? It was like a dream.

My husband agreed to see a paediatrician for our middle daughter. I researched available paediatricians. Waiting lists are long but persistence is my middle name, and I found a paediatrician, and presented my case. She agreed that my daughter showed traits related to autism and that further assessment was warranted.

Although my premonitions were validated, it was still a shock. Our world was slowly turning upside down. Based on the knowledge of my daughter probably being on the autism spectrum, my husband agreed to have the other two children visit the paediatrician, and we all went as a family. We had planned, in order of who we thought was a priority, to have our middle child assessed first, but the paediatrician threw us a curve ball. On hearing my presentations, she concluded our son required the most immediate support to manage his autism, with a high probability of a diagnosis of autism level 2. What's more, our youngest daughter also required more immediate support, also with a high probability of a diagnosis of autism level 2.

Both my husband and I walked out flabbergasted. I needed to talk. I had thought as much, but I was stunned. My husband had shut down. We had the kids with us and there was no opportunity for us to debrief. There was no talking to be had. Instead, we all went to Subway and the kids chose sandwiches, a treat in our home. Life for them was no different. Life for me was changing.

On the hour's drive home, I was planning. I was formulating. How on earth was I going to manage all of this? Three kids all with a possible diagnosis of autism level 2, and a diagnosis myself of autism level 2. I felt lost, burnt out, and honestly, frightened.

My first step was to rearrange appointments. I had previously booked an autism assessment for my middle daughter with a wait time of two weeks. We had already done the parent interview with the therapist. I rang the practice and pleaded to put my son in first. After some negotiating, they agreed. Right. Done. Next, I had to rebook my daughter. Not easy. I was also really conscious of pushing her appointment time back and how it looked to her. Thank goodness I have a background in counselling. I used all my strategies to validate her as an important person who hadn't just been shoved back for someone else - not an easy task!

Next, I had to think really carefully about my youngest. She is bouncy. She is a different learner from the older two children. For years my husband had been saying she has dyslexia, and for years I had been screaming that I had been experiencing difficulties managing her behaviour. To be frank, I was burning out. I found a therapist who specialised in autism and dyslexia and just to make sure, I asked her to include attention deficit disorder as well. The testing involved day trips down to Melbourne. For a full time business owner, and an autistic person who really thrives on routine, these trips were exhausting for me. The bigger picture was at stake though, and I would do whatever it took to support my child.

Our results came in. The older two children were confirmed with autism level 2. Our youngest child was diagnosed with autism level 2 with the addition of dyslexia. This meant four out of five of our family members were now identified as being on the autism spectrum. We had no extended family support. My parents-in-law refused to believe there was any issue and blamed it on the amount of time we let the kids use electronics. My father had gone years before and I had cut ties with my mother for self-protection. We were on our own to navigate the multitude of appointments, meltdowns and sensory overloads we now recognised as belonging to the world of autism. I felt for my husband.

Chapter 4
Rewind. Re-evaluating To Find A New Identity - Primary School

Fixation. A group of three girls all aged four. One girl, self-identifying as plump, fixated on these girls - a trait of female presentation of autism. I was good at kindergarten. I was so good, in fact, that my teacher told my mother that I had a really high level of general knowledge. My mother was proud. What my teacher didn't realise was how outcast I felt. Those three girls, in my mind, were beautiful, and I wanted to be friends with them, but I just didn't seem to be able to fit in. They were perfect, and me, I was nothing. A photo taken at the end of the year reflects this feeling like a magnifying glass. The girls are all standing together and I am just off to the side wearing a blue velvet jump suit. I felt so incredibly fat. I was four.

The next year it was suggested I repeat kindergarten, not because of my academic ability, but because of my age. This meant my brother was also going to be going to kinder with me. This didn't work in my mind. He fit in straight away. He found a mate and they are still friends to this day. I was, again, a loner. As a little girl, I couldn't fit. This time there were two girls. Beautiful girls. I wanted to play with them. They wouldn't let me in. No matter how much I tried, I felt different.

Lots of little girls are invited to parties. Lots of children have play dates. I can't recall being asked on a play date as a little girl. I can't recall party invitations. I would talk to my mother about how I felt. She would say I was just imagining things and that we can't all be friends with everyone. My loneliness fell on deaf ears.

After kindergarten it was time to transition to primary school. My brother stayed behind for another year in kindergarten. The beautiful girls were sent to the same school, and they were both put into my class. I sat with them, but they wouldn't let me play. What felt worse were the older kids in the class: I was put into a composite with both grade ones and preps. I wasn't sure about the older kids. When they came to talk to me, I clamped up. I had this belief that ages stick with ages. This meant all the kids the same age were meant to play together. I had a very regimented idea of how things should be done.

It also meant that the beautiful girls should stick with me. I had no ability to see beyond the two beautiful girls to the other 60 children in the classes, who might have been potential friends. All I saw were the girls who were already friends, and me on the outskirts.

I was lonely. I cried to my mother. What could she do? She spoke to the teacher and tried to intervene. I'm not sure what they discussed, but there were no changes. I remained fixated on the two girls and was crushed when they invited another girl into their friendship circle. I didn't understand.

My hearing was assessed, and I was found to be quite deaf in both ears due to wax build up. I needed grommets. At the same time, it was decided to remove my adenoids. I was operated on at the hospital where my mother worked as a weekend nurse. After the operation, I was sitting in hospital eating dinner. I was so full. My mother had ordered half a chicken for my dinner, and I was struggling to eat it all. A nurse came in and proclaimed astonishment that I was still eating. Although embarrassed, my response was simple: we weren't allowed to have dessert at home unless we ate all our dinner, so it was logical that I had to finish my plate before I was allowed to eat the jelly and ice-cream.

Follow up care was hard. I was to have regular hearing tests. The tests were noisy and would leave the buzzing reoccurring in my ears for weeks afterwards. Most of the time the noise was high pitched and would drown everything out. It was intense and difficult to handle.

My physical ability was assessed, and I was assessed as being uncoordinated and requiring intervention. The solution was to enrol me in a gym with kids three years younger than me. And include my brothers. I was mortified. Not only was this against the rules of ages staying in the same category, but I couldn't do the activities. My brothers could though, and they shimmied up those ropes easily, leaving me wondering what the hell was wrong with me and how on earth they could climb rope like that. To this day I still can't navigate monkey bars.

I was put into a physical activity group at school. All the unco kids had to leave class and do special activities. I never mastered them, no matter how much I tried.

So prep year was hard. The best thing I had discovered, though, was the world of books: I loved to read. I was good at reading. I was so good, I just slipped through the system and my academic ability was never questioned.

Grade One came. The teacher was beautiful. She was so skinny. She had a flat tummy. I was a fat plump kid. My father used to tell me I would end up like the side of a house and no one would love me. That meant this teacher was beautiful. I would run my hands over my fat belly at night and try and push it flat, to no avail. My memory of this teacher was her calling me the girl with the pink jeans on. I was mortified to be identified by the jeans I felt so fat in. I never wore those jeans again.

The kids in the class included the beautiful girls. Again, they wouldn't let me in. Again, in a class full of other kids, I never seemed to be able to see other kids, who might have been potential friends - all I focused on was getting these girls to accept me. Again, to no avail, so I remained lonely and fixated on a goal that at that time was unachievable.

Jump Rope for Heart was promoted at school. This was a whole school activity. Every physical education class was focused on jumping with a skipping rope. Every kid at break time was practising jumping with skipping ropes. I couldn't do it. I was mortified. Again, I cried to my mother. She just pulled me out of school the day of the big skipping competition. It wasn't until Grade Five that I actually learned to jump that damn rope.

Around this time, I had started developing regular stomachaches. My father said I was faking it. My mother dragged me to the doctor, and scans and tests were done, but they found nothing. The stomachaches hurt though, and I had no way of getting rid of them. I just had to put up with them.

My father; well, together we were just a lost cause. He was becoming more aggressive. My mother became distant, and at times she would run away, leaving me with my father and brothers. This wasn't ideal. She was the only ally I had in my court, and the only believer of the stomachaches.

In Grade Two the Cabbage Patch Kid doll was popular. Every kid had one. I didn't. This meant I couldn't play with them at school. I still had no friends. One day, towards the end of the fad, my father took me to the toyshop. He told me to choose a Cabbage Patch Kid. Oh, my goodness, I was thrilled! Finally after all this time I had a Cabbage Patch Kid. I proudly took it to school the next day. A week later the My Child doll was in and Cabbage Patch Kids were out. What was I going to do with this $80 doll I didn't even really like? I wasn't a player. I had no imagination when it came to pretend play. Organised play I could follow. It had structure. Pretend play had no rules and I wasn't sure what to do. So the Cabbage Patch Kid got shoved aside.

Routines and structure meant safety. I knew what to expect. Growing up in a Catholic family meant that every Sunday morning at 9am we would attend Mass. We would sit in the front row as a family, and sometimes I even had a role, which made me feel important and also helped to make a boring ceremony a little more bearable.

I was sent to a Catholic school for my education, which meant that Grade Three was all about the First Communion. I had a vision of how this was supposed to be. Too bad I looked so fat in my white First Communion dress. I felt just awful. The highlight of the day was seeing all my cousins; I loved that. There was also amazing food! The downside was my father telling me to stop eating, I was getting too fat. My perception of the God-like day was squashed and I ended up in tears. I was not supposed to get yelled at on the God Day. I was supposed to be protected. It didn't happen.

Finally, finally, finally the beautiful girls let me in. Grade Five was different: I had a friendship circle. After so many years I finally felt like I belonged and was accepted. I still had to psychoanalyse every move everyone made to make sure I was ok, but I was accepted! I played netball, and I was good at it. In fact, I was very good at it! I could jump a rope. In fact, I was good at that too.

Academically I was intelligent. Things on that front were going well; and just in time.

Things on the home front were unravelling. My father and mother were getting worse together. My stomachaches stopped and I was experiencing headaches. They hurt - ranging from mild to severe, I was suffering with headaches every day now. My father said I was faking it. My mother dragged me to the doctor. Scans and tests were done. The result: nothing.

We were never quite told, but adopted the silent approach for what was happening at home. My parents were abusive. My father was periodically aggressive and we never knew when he would blow; but boy, when he blew up, he blew up. At one time I was so scared I called the police. My grandfather bailed him out from being charged by the police, saying he didn't want his daughter married to a jailbird. It is really difficult to provide evidence for emotional abuse.

My mother would confide in me; I was her support. As a child, it was too much for me to handle. I had to protect her from him. This developed into a triangle relationship, with me in the middle. My role in the family was to become the scapegoat for all the bad things.

In Grade Six this became magnified. The teacher played favourites. She had this amazing idea of putting twenty-five different activities up on a chart under the theme of sheep. I loved it! An example of integrated learning at its finest! I wrote a song, including lyrics and sheet music. I showed it to my organ teacher. She corrected all my mistakes. I never wrote again. I did twenty-four of those tasks. I was so proud. My teacher was proud - of another student. She praised the student for completing twenty of the tasks. But I had completed twenty-four. I didn't understand. I was playing by her rules but they weren't clear for me.

This teacher would go off tap. She would lose her temper often, and I didn't feel safe. My classmates would get together and talk about a boycott. I would sit in class when she yelled and imagine just getting up and walking home. I really wanted to. I just didn't, though. I couldn't work out how to play her game.

I was also getting fatter. My chest was developing and I hated it. I would wear really big tee-shirts to try and hide my chest. I was also experiencing severe pain in my nipples; every time I caught a chill they hurt like hell. They burned and anything that touched them caused so much pain. I didn't tell anyone. I was so embarrassed.

I got my period. I hated it. Squishy stupid thing. I felt so irritated before it. I would be on overload. Everything was too much: it was too loud, it was too bright, it was too consuming. My temper would fray. Every month I would be fighting with every member of my family. I was feeling so alone. And then I would get my period. Somehow, I had to navigate back into everyone's good books as my moods settled down. My headaches continued.

I felt safe at primary school. I knew the routine. I knew every person in my year level. I went to church there every week. I was known. I was the good girl who even played the organ at Mass. We were regarded as the perfect family. My mother was on the Parish Committee and the School Council. Then came the transition to high school.

Chapter 5
Rewind. Re-evaluating To Find A New Identity - High School

I didn't cope. My route to school was an hour long. I had to get a bus, then a train, and then a bus again. I panicked. Every night I had anxiety I would miss the bus. I would set my alarm and wake up in a panic before the alarm. I walked to the bus stop and would be in a panic until the bus arrived. It never once entered my mind that if I missed the bus, I could just get the next one. I had to get the right bus at the right time. The same with the train. I had to get the right train at the right time. The amount of panic all of this caused was tremendous.

I was also aware of my cheeks wobbling on the bus. I felt fat in my uniform, and it was heavy and scratchy. I thought I looked awful. My cheeks wobbling confirmed how awful I was, and I would grit my teeth together to stop them from wobbling. This was to become important to me later on.

My friends were going to a different school, and the one friend in our group who was going to my school was the one person I didn't get along with so well. This meant I was pretty much on my own. For the first year of Year Seven I was lost. The friend had made other friends. In my rules we were supposed to remain friends. She was not following the rules. I was confused.

By the end of Year Seven I became friends with another girl. She had a best friend too, but I was able to get in. There were a few other girls in the group as well, but I was mostly fixated on the main girl. The two of us would later encourage each other to take some not so healthy risks.

My parents separated when I was in Year Eight. I was mortified. For years I had been begging my mother to leave my father. I had prayed to God. I had begged God. I had done some pretty wild deals with God, all to no avail. When they finally separated, I broke down. My family were supposed to be the epiphany of

Godliness. We were perfect, in a way. Suddenly we were dirty. No one else in my friendship circle had parents who had separated. How was I going to share this information?

For my brothers it was a different story. Every second weekend, all of my three brothers were invited to Dad's flat. He said he didn't want me there. He said he was ashamed to have me there. I felt the knife of rejection twisting in deep. Every time they came back, they had boxes of cereal with them. It was Flintstones Pebbles, a sugary cereal. For us kids this was a huge big deal - we had never had sugary cereal before - but he didn't bring me any. I was rejected. Severely. I knew that we had our issues, but this was out and out rejection. My mother ignored it. I became more aggressive.

I retreated into my own hellhole. I was trying to make sense of all these different messages I was receiving. I was still having anxiety about getting the bus on time. I was becoming the queen of masking! On the outside I was bright and bubbly, albeit a little eccentric at times. I was called loud, and told to use my inside voice on numerous occasions.

On the inside I was fragile and frightened. I questioned everything and had little trust in anyone. My mother continued to say I blamed everyone but myself. She told me that all my teachers said I would blame them. Me, I just wanted to be accepted. My father didn't accept me, and my mother needed me as a confidante, not as a daughter. I felt blamed, unwanted and misunderstood. And I was still battling those headaches.

One night my mother had the local priest over for tea. This man, to me, was a God figure. He had been at my First Communion. He had been at my Confirmation. He was a figure of authority to be revered.

This night was to be a turning point in my life. For the last six months I had been trying to diet, and I wasn't very good at it. I learned how to count calories and had myself down to a lettuce leaf for most of the day but would lose it after a few days. The night the priest came over I learned how to vomit my meal. I discovered the power of being able to let go all my thoughts and feelings. This gave me an amazing feeling of control and power. I felt empty and yet elated at the same time. Surely, I was meant to do this. We had the man of God in our house and I was raised as a good Catholic. Surely this was a sign that God wanted me to live my life this way? I was so grateful to have found a path to wellness and love. I followed this path faithfully and with dedication.

I found my routine. Eat, purge, eat, purge. The headaches stopped! The stomach pains at that time were long gone. The only issue was I became so good at it, everything else had to go by the wayside. My locus of control was out of control.

Around this time, I became unruly. The emotional outbursts were happening more frequently, and there were times when I would completely trash my parents 'room. No one ever said anything. I was getting tired, and I started skipping school. No one said anything. What people did say, though, was how good I looked! I was losing weight, fast. I was in control. I no longer had to deal with any emotion and I was feeling liberated. Scared, but liberated.

I developed a full-blown eating disorder. I was treated as an eating disorder patient. I was given cognitive behavioural therapy (CBT) and outpatient care. I progressed really well: I understood the logic of CBT and was able to apply the method. The only issue, though, was that my parents were still out of control. My father was in and out of my mother's life and consequently mine. He still refused to see me. That was suiting me fine. Then my mother decided it was time for them to reunite. I didn't cope.

Autism burnout. I was chronically exhausted. My previously high academic standards were now reduced to grades of Ds and Fs. I had lost all interest in life and was experiencing a reduced tolerance to situations. Autism burnout is described by Raymaker et al. (2021) as an experience lasting for more than three months occurring during a time of life transition. On reflection, this was the first occurrence I have experienced of autistic burnout. I had lost all hope.

My mother accepted my father home. They reunited. I moved out that very night. I was fifteen years old, and I just packed my bag and left. My mind was unable to readjust to the situation. I was fixated on the pain they caused me. I was aware of the sudden shock of my father's raised voice and the deep pain I experienced as I had consoled my mother. My reserves were empty. I had to escape. In the words of Miserandino (2003), I was out of spoons.

There was one highlight, however: I had become fixated on a bloke. Five and a half years older than me, this bloke was my target. At one of the only parties I had been to, I had met this bloke, the older brother of the host. He was a stoner. He had showed a little interest in me. For a girl who had been told she was too fat and no one would love her - to paraphrase the words of my father - this was a miracle, and I believed I had to hold onto this relationship. So I chased him. Half the time he was too stoned to even notice me. I didn't give up though: I rang ten times a day, I walked to his house - over ten kilometres to and from his house - to be frank, I was relentless. To be frank, I never even considered whether or not I actually liked him. That never even entered my mind.

I had left home. I was trying to go to school and work to pay rent at the same time. I had hooked up with the bloke and was becoming the queen of self-medication. So I quit school. I am so grateful to have autistic determination! Somehow, I survived because I had a target.

Chapter 6
Leaving School and Entering a Different Domain - Eating Disorder City Here I Come!

I worked. I saved my money. I was a good budgeter. Every month I caught the train from Ringwood to Mitcham to hand over my hard-earned cash to the real estate agent to keep a roof over my head. The real estate agent took my money every month. Every month I paid my electricity bill; every month I paid my water bill; every month I paid my phone bill. I was sixteen years old.

Food bills: that was another issue. Every couple of months I would put on my autistic masking skills and pretend to St Vincent De Paul that all was good. They would randomly drop over and hand me a $100 bill. This meant I could eat for a while. I also received a box of veggies on my door step every fortnight. I was a survivor, at this stage an unknown survivor of autism with a diagnosed eating disorder.

I got stuck. My fixation on this bloke was fierce, and I stayed with him for five years. Together we had a tumultuous relationship made more confused by self-medication and traumas. It was not healthy.

Ever a survivor, I took a job as an apprentice chef. I was obsessed with food. I read food magazines. I read cookbooks. I studied recipes. I made cut outs to formulate my own recipe books. I had a diagnosed eating disorder. Food was my obsession.

I worked a full year as an apprentice chef, and I became thinner and thinner. The more I worked, the more obsessed I became with food. The more obsessed I became, the less I ate. Finally, my body started giving up.

I was admitted to an eating disorder hospital. I had done it! I was the best! I had made it all the way to hospital and I was so proud. I just couldn't seem to find my way back though. I was fixated on kilojoules and the number on the scale. It had to be as low as it could possibly get. Unfortunately, there is no food that has zero kilojoules.

This was an issue. I would wander for hours after working as a chef analysing every food for the least kilojoules. I would weigh myself multiple times a day watching that number go lower. My moods were dependant on those figures and controlling those figures. I had taught myself this game. I knew the rules. I was now being asked to give it up?! No way!

In hospital you conform to their rules. You have to play their games. If you do, you are a good girl. If you don't, you are defiant and a troublemaker. I had my own rules, and my rules didn't match their rules. I was in trouble. I tried my best, I really did, but the logic that I was told from the nurses and the dietician didn't match with my own logic. Still, I agreed to try.

I was discharged to live with my mother. At this time my parents had permanently separated and I was now in my teens. I started seeing a psychiatrist at the same time twice a week. This became a new ritual. I finally dumped the boyfriend. I was on my own, in the basement of my mother's house.

Routine. What is routine and what is obsession? My routines became obsessional. I had to keep clean. I washed my body twenty-four times each day. My skin started becoming inflamed. The floor had to be swept in a strategic way at least four times a day. No skerrick of dust was allowed to be seen on that wooden floor. My exercise structure had to be morning and night, a set route for a specific amount of time. Breakfast was the same every day, at the same time. Lunch was the same every day, at the same time. Dinner was the same every day, at the same time. Any deviation would cause an outburst. The evenings were times to relax. Only then could I indulge in eight apples and take pride in feeling full.

This routine was, to say the least, exhausting. There was no possibility of a social life. My family ridiculed my behaviour and told me I was faking it. My mother was at her wits' end struggling with her own stuff. I was on my own, with no ability to work or study. All my spoons were reserved for the twice weekly trip into town to see the psychiatrist and the other behaviours that made up the day, some of which I'm too ashamed to mention.

Something had to give, and give it did. I landed back in hospital again. This time I was more defiant and didn't want to be there. I already knew the drill. I snuck out for walks. I played the piano and sang at the top of my voice. I hid food. I confided in a nurse that I felt uncomfortable with a male patient sleeping near me. And then the ultimate - the lead clinician told me my weight, in front of a panel of 24 professionals. I really flipped my lid. He kickstarted again the game I had been so careful to stop on my first admission. The scales became obsessional. He really had no idea of the danger he was doing to me and dismissed my aggressive outburst as an act of defiance.

I was discharged, this time for an admission as a day patient at another hospital. This was a group program. I was told I was lucky to be in the program. I was expected to behave, and I was expected to get along with the other girls in the group. The only issue was I didn't understand them. My anxiety at being made to catch public transport and not walk the few kilometres to the hospital was through the roof after being made to sit all day. My anxiety at being forced to have double protein, full fat yoghurts and snacks was displayed as aggression. I wasn't able to conform.

I managed the best I could. Sometimes I just had to leave. In the social outing, watching *Saving Private Ryan*, I left after the violent scene. It was overload. I was reprimanded the next day. I was forced to close my eyes and have my eyelashes tinted. I was freaked out! I silently threw the double proteins in the bin. The group confronted me. I was accused of being sneaky and lying. I was not a team player. They had bonded and I hadn't. I had the lowest weight and I was most defiant. I didn't fit. They made friends and I didn't. I couldn't work out why.

This is autism at its finest. Every activity I undertook was to alleviate anxiety. I had suffered throughout my childhood from social anxiety and social miscommunication. I wasn't able to understand the rules of friendship and would become fixated on one group and one group only. My family were unresponsive to my needs and I had no language to represent what I was feeling. Added to this was the ongoing monthly aggression which was still occurring, causing sensory overload and constant periods of isolation. I didn't fit the model to cure my eating disorder.

So I left. I discharged myself against the wisdom of the hospital staff and enrolled in a course at the local TAFE. Here, I fitted. I had a story. I was now twenty-one years old and visibly anorexic. The study, though, was a saviour. It provided routine. It provided structure. It provided knowledge and I was able to fixate on something else, the meaning of behaviour. I was fascinated.

Chapter 7
Growing Up – Moving On

I coped really well for the first six months. Then it became a little too hard and I started skipping class to go for walks. I landed back in hospital again for a two-week stint. This was my last admission for an eating disorder, I am proud to say. I had found another fixation: study.

For the next four years I was a full-time student at TAFE. I studied Youthwork, Welfare, Community Development and Visual Arts. I was safe and comfortable. However, study does end, and the time came for me to enter the workforce.

I'd dabbled in work a few times. I always seemed to end up in conflict. I had my way of doing things and what I was seeing just didn't always seem right. I also saw so many breaches of ethics. I didn't understand this. It caused so much conflict in my mind and I would spend countless hours analysing the events over and over. I had to learn strategies for handling these situations.

I had met the man who was to be my husband by this stage. This time, the relationship was different, and there was no fixation. We entered the relationship on a more equal level, even though I brought along with me years of rejection, trauma and the tail end of an eating disorder. He just accepted me and it was this acceptance that helped me to grow.

I chewed his ear off. Every single night. I analysed. He reassured. I re-analysed. He re-reassured. To be frank, it was exhausting for both of us. I was also suffering from a diagnosed disorder of social anxiety and body dysmorphia and was self-medicating. The PMDD was still rearing its ugly head every month but at that stage we had no language for it.

I wasn't cut out for the welfare workforce. I was bullied. I tried to be assertive. The women wouldn't let me in. The young people I was working with were in pain. I didn't know how to help. So I continued to chew my husband's ear off.

We both agreed time out. I started studying a Graduate Diploma of Education. My husband was a teacher and we agreed it would get me out of the pain of youthwork and into a productive job. So once again I studied, and I coped really well. I got good marks. I enjoyed my study.

It didn't come without its challenges, though. As an autistic person I am trained to read situations. This helps me predict what is safe and when I need to be on my guard. I am not always correct, and in fact in some circumstances I have been so far off that I have missed many opportunities for connection. Sometimes though, I don't listen. This happened a few times on placements for my Graduate Diploma. I saw things that are reportable offences in schools, but I shut my mouth, afraid. I was bullied by my supervisor. I had no recourse to handle this. It shattered me. I kept going and ended up graduating with an A grade average.

I married my husband and we had an amazing little boy. I loved being a mummy, but I had lost my structure. I didn't fit into the mums' group I was put into. I was too paranoid and I couldn't relax. Small talk has never been my thing: I don't see the point. I also had so much baggage that I was sure they could see I was essentially a bad person; after all, I had been accumulating evidence to confirm this throughout my whole life. I floundered in this group.

We also had a next-door neighbour who loved to rev his engine. He also liked bass music. I was agitated. I would fixate on this sound, and wherever I went in the house, I suffered. I would become aggressive. I had no language at that time to understand I was on sensory overload.

So we moved. We took the plunge and moved to the country. We left behind our family and friends. Most of the friends were my husband's; I had struggled for years to fit in with his friends. With my own, they were thin and more easily managed as acquaintances. It took all my energy to socialise and without the aid of a bottle or two, I would struggle.

The best thing about being a new mum was that the PMDD disappeared. For ten years we lived without the mood fluctuations.

Yes, I would become anxious at social events, but it was manageable. I had a role. I was a mother and could hide behind my children. My whole focus now was on my children.

I wasn't a player; I was a doer. I would do things for them, but not with them. I could buy them toys but had no imagination to help me play with them. I would buy them craft packs but even with my diploma in visual arts could not seem to find the creativity to use the items. I was very good at keeping the house tidy though and the clothes put away. I was a great coffee mum, visiting a coffee shop on my own with the kids in tow. This was some semblance of what constituted normality, and I strove to fit into a neurotypical world.

I took them to playgroups. It backfired. I tried, but I struggled to socialise and afterwards I was drained. My spoons were depleted, but I kept on trying. I was put into another mothers' group. It flopped. My child was six months older and at that stage there is a massive difference between children's developments. I was striving to fit in, not stand out.

Again, I immersed myself in study. I believed I was struggling to control depression. I was enjoying the study, and I was finding studying yoga to be helpful. The study was structured. It was tangible and I was putting it into practice. After this, I studied Ayurveda. I learned so much about food. My control was food. Ayurveda showed me freedom through education. I lapped up everything I could.

Studying Ayurveda was hard, and I had to travel. This took me out of my comfort zone and away from the familiarity of my family. I stayed away for long stretches. I couldn't understand why I was not fitting in with my peers. We were all fascinated by the same topic. I was practising it in my life. Instead, I was called 'high energy' and 'ever ready battery'. I struggled to make sense of these remarks against the backdrop of study. It is only now that I see my autistic fixation is more apparent when I am passionate about something. I become fascinated in a topic. Only now I have learned, through necessity, that not everyone has the same level of energy and passion that I have. Knowing I had autism earlier might have helped me avoid this confusion.

Around this time my mother decided to sell her house in Mitcham and build a town house. We invited her to live with us, in our granny flat, during the build. Big mistake.

Scenario. Take one undiagnosed autistic female adult. Add a mother who has been a victim of domestic violence, with her own history of parental abuse. Now stir. It does not work. My mother came in with her ideas. I came with mine. My carefully carved routine was criticised. We had bowl food. I was accused of training her to eat at set times. She left wine glasses lying around. I lost track of where my children were. It didn't work. Even more than that, I was accustomed to picking up her every tone, and I would flinch at the tongue click. A look from her would send me into a spin. This arrangement lasted twelve months before it was decided she would be better suited in a rental.

From there, family support went out the window. We rarely, if ever, had visits from the in-laws. We went down when we could and when I had the energy. My brothers rarely, if ever, visited our place. Our connections became fragmented and my children were losing any relationship they once had with their cousins.

Family dynamics in my family of origin had never been great anyway. My father had long since left my life, twenty years earlier, and he had hooked up with another Polish broad and her kids. We had our battles over my grandfather's will and he tried to personally attack me. I had taken him to court years before for verbal aggression, with the intention of obtaining a restraining order, to no avail. He had me arrested for taking my things from his house. There was no love lost there, just dormant pain.

My target was to try to keep family relations with my mother and brother. It just wasn't working though. The more I tried, the more I was rejected. My language wasn't their language. My obsession with study was misunderstood, and I was classified as cold and uncaring. On the contrary, I couldn't have cared more. It hurt, like hell, on a cycle of repeat until the day I decided to press stop - permanently.

Chapter 8
What is Autism?

Autism is classed as a neurodevelopmental disability defined as persistent deficits in the areas of social communication and interaction to include social reciprocity, nonverbal communication and skills in developing, maintaining and understanding relationships. A formal diagnosis of autism, as defined by the Diagnostic and Statistical Manual five, (DSM IV), includes the addition of restricted and repetitive patterns of behaviour, interests or activities (Azizi., 2015).

Autism is defined as a spectrum. This means there is agreement on a range of different manifestations of the disability that affect individuals at varying degrees. Severity levels, ranging from level one as the lowest level to level three as the highest level, are designed to categorise the disability as a tool to guide the levels of interventions required (Hodges et al., 2019).

Autism as a spectrum is a different way of viewing the disability. Stereotypes, such as Dustin Hoffman's character in the movie *Rain Man* (1988), have brought to the public attention a particular image of autism. Sheldon Cooper in the sitcom *The Big Bang Theory* (2007-2019) portrays the features of autism in his regimented behaviours, monotone delivery and fixative interests. Furthermore, the stereotype of autism is seen in Sam in the sitcom *Atypical* (2017-present).

All of these characters are male. All of these characters represent a stereotypical image of autism: monotone delivery, lack of empathy and obsessional behaviour. The characters also serve to reinforce the stereotype that males are more likely to receive a diagnosis than females.

What these characters do well is increase awareness that autism is not restricted to childhood. Children grow up. With them, so does the autism. Current services are overwhelmed with children and waiting lists are long. Access to adult friendly services is not readily available.

Growing up in the 1970s, I was a child who met all of my developmental milestones. I was bright, my kindergarten teacher referred to my general knowledge level as high, I read well, and I required minimal academic support. I did not meet the image of the Sheldons in the world.

Growing up in the 2020s, my children all met their developmental milestones. In fact, my mother lived with us for a year when my son was little, and she is a trained and experienced maternal and child health nurse - and she missed all the signs and symptoms of autism in both me and the children. My children all learned to read well and were academically bright, with the exception of my youngest child. She was still sent to school, however, as she was assessed by her kindergarten teacher as meeting the requirements for social learning skills for school. The stereotypes threw us off guard. We were not ready, based on these stereotypes.

Enter Dana in the sitcom *Superstore* (2015-2021): a notable portrayal of autism which sent the social media world of autistic adults into a flurry. A female representation of autism. Love her or hate her, she was accepted by her peers. The portrayal of Rebecca Bunch in *My Crazy ExGirlfriend* (2015-2019) highlights a refreshingly comical, at times dark, tale of fixation and addiction. This sitcom is not only cleverly written as a musical, it also provides creative flair. What becomes intriguing is the disclosure of Rebecca's diagnosis of borderline personality disorder in season four.

Having been given a diagnosis of borderline personality disorder, I was shellshocked. This was difficult to comprehend. Was I domineering? Was this a portrayal of what I was like? Research in autism and borderline personality disorder by Dudas et al. (2019) suggests an overlap between the two disorders. Furthermore, a diagnosis based on an outward display of behaviours may negate altogether the inward attitude that is commonly present in autism (Pearson et al., 2021). Many of the stereotypes of autistic behaviour are displays, or lack of, behaviours associated with autism.

The external and internal turmoil of borderline personality disorder is regarded as an inability to regulate emotions leading to confusion in role identity and expertise in manipulation. Extreme emotions can be seen in both borderline personality disorder and autism, and it takes a skilled clinician to differentiate between the two. For what purpose? I remember my aunty asking why I was chasing a diagnosis. My response was simple. To understand myself. As a recipient of BPD diagnosis, I was medicated. The treatment of choice was DBT. I researched DBT. In fact, I spent hours researching DBT. It is expensive. I researched health insurance companies. In fact, I spent hours researching health insurance companies. When eventually I joined a DBT group, it only served to validate the internal feelings that I was rotten to the inner core. I was kicked out of the group and my money was refunded. Why? Because it is the incorrect treatment for a person with autism.

Recall that the diagnosis of autism may include difficulties in social cognition. The experience of group therapy in DBT is essential to practise skills. The modules of DBT are designed to encourage emotional regulation, based on skilling the client in tolerating stressors to live in the moment and make decisions from the rational mind. Activities such as flushing ice-cold water on the face are designed to shock the client to re-regulate and come back to the moment. This is taught alongside individual therapy. The group-based component of DBT was confronting. I had minimal skills in social communication and at that moment in time was extremely vulnerable. Combined with an inability to 'read 'the group as a whole, and the sensory stimulation of video and noise, the treatment program was unsuitable for a presentation of autism without additional support.

The importance of a correct diagnosis is also evident in the treatment of eating disorders. My experience of group therapy, both as an inpatient and as an outpatient, demonstrates the turmoil a client with a dual diagnosis of autism and eating disorder can experience. Group therapy demands a reciprocal response. In her manual on group therapy for eating disorders, McBride (2012) suggests there are three features for effective group therapy: understanding the personality of the group members, interaction between individual group members and interaction of the group as a whole system. Again, recall that the diagnosis of autism defines difficulties in social cognition: a person with autism cannot contribute effectively with the group process without additional supports. This was evidenced by my inability to form relationships with other group members in hospital. My behaviours to reduce anxiety were misconstrued as devious and deliberate.

Understanding autism helps to create an environment of understanding. The core features of autism - deficiency in social communication, repetitive behaviours and restricted behaviours - can be further understood by evaluating the meanings beyond the behaviours. Sensory overload, sensation seeking or difficulties in communication may be understood from the individual context as they materialise, resulting in better management - as opposed to trying to fix something that ain't broke.

Chapter 9
Adult Late Diagnosis Autism

Imagine spending your entire life on a search for wellness. There is an inkling something is wrong but you just can't put your finger on it because really, you feel fine. It just seems like there is bad luck, always.

As a child, I knew there was something wrong. I was aware our family weren't normal. My father did things that were strange, and which I couldn't understand. His words to me were just awful. I already felt alone, and compounded with the confusion caused by abuse from a caregiver, the message a child develops is that there is something wrong with them. Stomachaches, headaches and later anorexia were external displays of internalised anxiety.

A child is helpless really to learn about life without the support of their parents, and the norms that are developed set the stage for the formation of social identity. Pearson et al. (2021) discuss the development of the social identity based on social learning theory. Social learning theory proposes that our sense of self is developed from the environment and the context we find ourselves in. The way we are received by those around us affects our perception of ourselves. A child who receives messages that she is different, abnormal or dysfunctional may begin to develop a self-perception of deficit. This reflects my story.

Throughout my childhood and into early adulthood I worked with the medical model understanding of mental health. The medical model follows a deficit model to identify symptoms that are problematic and provides suggestions for improvement. One of the biggest misdemeanours of our time was the fluctuation of the diagnostic criteria forming the framework for the autistic model. To be frank, the idea of me having autism as a child would have been laughable at the time. I presented as a bright and intelligent child with a high level of general knowledge coming from a good Catholic family. What wasn't seen were the challenges with social communication, repetitive behaviours, high levels of anxiety and slow developing motor skills that are commonly recognised traits of autism. In addition, I was female.

So, what has happened to create a sudden increase in autism? The first change was the re-evaluation of what constitutes autism. Between the 1980s and 1990s the criteria for an autism diagnosis was expanded (Pelicano et al., 2020). To make it more confusing, Stagg et al. (2019) suggest the changes to diagnostic benchmarks may have resulted in a section of the population remaining undiagnosed. Coining the term 'the lost generation', McDonald (2020) suggests that there is growing awareness that being female has been an additional barrier to a diagnosis of autism, and as people are ageing, the awareness of social barriers is resulting in a new wave of adults seeking a diagnosis or self-diagnosing.

This lost generation of people, who are being diagnosed late in life, are having to deal with a whole new way of understanding themselves, and their past experiences. Services for adults with autism are slim at their best. How, then, does one navigate the world with this newfound information which rocks the core of identity? When I was trying to recover from anorexia nervosa I wrote. My journal was my best friend. I literally poured my heart into the pages of my journal, and this helped me argue with the voices in my head. This ended up being a published book and I hope my thoughts have helped others who have experienced the trauma of eating disorders. What my journal highlights for me is the level of anxiety I suffered, and my approach to regulating that anxiety. I also suffered - well, still do suffer - from a very low self-esteem. I generally analyse to the nth degree every move, action and behaviour to make sure everything is ok.

I used to debrief with my mother. Now my husband has this role and, in some ways, talking with him has replaced the endless writing in my journals. These behaviours are comparable to Molloy et al.'s (2004) discussion of meaning-making in the act of trying to take control and present new narratives to make sense of the past and the present. The result is continual evaluation, to make meaning and perhaps increase self-confidence on reflection of social performance and self-perceived performance. This is exhausting to say the least!

Not surprisingly, I felt isolated. These were very obsessive behaviours and the more I was able to talk and reflect, the more control I perceived I would have, to be able to react appropriately to situations, or to understand whether I was at fault in situations. I was sometimes truly desperate for my husband to understand to the full extent what I was experiencing. Having a diagnosis of autism now has allowed us to become aware of where the communication difficulties exist and take steps to reprocess. This comes from a very deep, long-term place. Many people with autism experience difficulties with isolation, unemployment and poor mental health because the core problem has not been identified and there has been a lifetime of mental health resulting from perceived deficits from living in a neurotypical world.

For so many years, in fact for most of my life, I was searching for answers to help me solve my idiosyncrasies. I had this yellow book. It was my cut and paste book. One year I went to Confest, an alternative festival full of natural therapies and a smorgasbord of ideologies for wellbeing. I was in heaven. I would examine the workshop board every day and night meticulously, looking for the 'right 'therapy that could act like the magic pill. I would record my experiences and analyse the availability of services in my area to help me pursue this new answer. Classic autism! The only problem was nothing really worked.

So, armed with the new knowledge that there is something developmentally different about you, how do you cope? The very core of who you thought you were, and who you were told you were, has changed. And let's face it, getting a diagnosis is hard enough really.

I grieved. I was angry. I was sad. I felt like I was an imposter. The title of autism was a relief. It meant in a way I could stop expending all that energy on trying to fit into a world that I was not a part of. My therapist and I would have many discussions about my expectations for relationships. She would ask me what it would be like if I allowed myself to only have one or two friends instead of holding on to the need to have a whole netball team of friends to choose from. I always fought her on this. Having autism for me meant that it was ok to be on my own and enjoy writing this book. It was ok to really enjoy writing assignments for my psychology course. My self-image as an outgoing person was re-examined and I truly had to admit that I loved reading psychology reports and sitting in my jammies listening to the rain with a big cup of chai on a Sunday afternoon. I had to admit that this was actually me in my element. And it made me happy.

What was really confronting was the immense amount of questioning I did. That imposter syndrome is a bugger. I had previously worked with people who had autism. I had been their teacher. Suddenly I belonged to this group? No way. For months, actually maybe a year, I would ask my husband, 'Do I really have autism?' 'Yes,' he would say. Every session with my therapist I would ask her to validate whether I had autism. 'Are we really going back there again?' she would ask. 'Yes,' I would say. 'Yes Sarah, you really do have autism,' was her weekly reply.

Newly diagnosed or self-identified members of the autism community commonly experience imposter syndrome. The whole world has suddenly tipped upside down; or there is validation of a gnawing feeling of difference. When I was diagnosed, I told my family, and I got back some pretty nasty responses. My brother was downright abusive. My mother read through my multitude of professional reports and then later sent me a long letter denying the diagnosis and blaming it on my past use of self-medication and a fall I had when I was six years old. This situation is called gaslighting. The responses from my family made me question myself. Did I really have autism? Maybe I faked it? Maybe I really am rotten to the core and they are right, I'm a fake.

This is a scenario I read over and over again on social media. Adults who are newly diagnosed tell their family of origin. The family disagrees. The person experiences gaslighting - a situation where the newly diagnosed person is forced to re-question their diagnosis again and again, sometimes almost causing them to feel insane! This, I learned, is classified as a form of mental abuse. To take control of a life that is now viewed through the glasses of autism, sometimes the family need to be let go of. This in itself is a traumatic experience that causes a big bump in the road to self-acceptance. And it hurts.

Not only was I advised, in the end, to cut my ties with my family of origin, I had to process the grief and anger I felt towards them. I was 43 years old at the time of diagnosis. Half my life was gone! My life felt like a lie!

It was time to re-evaluate and reconfigure a new identity. How do you do that when the experiences you have had to date have been violation on violation of trust, and you haven't had the ability to understand why? The first step I took was to re-evaluate how much I did. Actually, that was pretty easy. I had come to a point where I was so wrung out that it wasn't really that difficult to stop being overloaded.

I quit being a member of the school council at the children's school. My expectations of myself included being involved with the kids' school to show I cared. For me, this was torture. I couldn't remember anyone's name. We transitioned to online meetings due to Covid; I was a whiz with Zoom, having used it myself for teaching over the past five years, but the school used Teams and this was another system altogether, which just didn't make sense for me. The council also used drop box for information sharing. To this day I am still a gumby with drop box! This was pressure and I resigned.

The second thing I did was to withdraw. Literally. My puff had run out. I had myself a break socially. Maybe a little too much. I joined Facebook groups and immersed myself in the world of neurodiversity. I learned so much and am still learning.

Through these associations I learned about the concept of masking. I was always so proud of my ability to camouflage into any group. My first boyfriend was quite frankly a criminal self-medicator, and we lived for a time with his family. His mother chose not to work and spent most of her money on bingo. It was great when she won because then that meant we would have some food and the electricity bill would be paid again. To this day I hate cold showers! I was proud of my ability to adapt to their living standards, having come from an all-girls Catholic school. I bought a surfy top when I had a boyfriend who was into surfing. I could hold my own when it came to sitting outside at the Perth YMCA talking small talk with people who I later learned were homeless. I could adapt my conversation to work fairly productively with the young people in my jobs as a youth worker. I tried my hardest to fit in socially with my peers. I would be exhausted at the end of a coffee date, trying to hold conversation and frantically pre-think where I could lead the discussion.

This is masking. Maybe people saw my red face or observed I would trip over my words in Team meetings. Little did they know my heart would be racing and my little voice would be rehearsing over and over and over. Masking is hard. It is hiding the true identity. For me it was living in fear that I would be discovered as a fraud.

One year I decided to volunteer at a yoga event with a Yoga Association. Now, I love yoga. It really did change my life, probably because I had been suffering with undiagnosed and unrecognised anxiety manifesting as aggression and confusion throughout my life to date. I was very enthusiastic about yoga. It gave me a break from my mind. My body was directed into movement and for that time period I didn't have to think. It also helped me to breathe, which was a tool I took off the mat into daily life. I had also become very enthusiastic about Ayurveda. This was regarded as the sister science to yoga and I saw a connection that was apparent. I had suffered so badly with an eating disorder that learning what I ate and how I ate therapeutically had a powerful influence on my yoga. This was applied Ayurveda in action.

So enthusiastic was I that I was guided to write a course in Ayurveda Yoga. At the time the concept was relatively new in Australia and I experienced a lot of criticism. Unfortunately, I was unable to read the feedback properly and I was so enthusiastic about what I had researched that any criticism was taken personally. I was confused. Volunteering for the yoga event was difficult. I had already come in as a late volunteer and wasn't sure if my delay in acceptance was personal or business. The group were using drop box for communication. The dreaded drop box. I still can't work out how to navigate this system! On the day of the event, I was a bundle of nerves. It was in town and I was from regional Victoria. This meant an overnight stay. I was well out of my comfort zone. The trip down was full of unexpected roadworks and I arrived buzzed and scattered. Everyone was busy and I just couldn't get a read on the situation. On day three I fell down a hole. My head hurt. I had to leave, knowing if I didn't go then, I wouldn't make it home. Halfway home I had to pull over and sleep. On arrival at home, I crawled to bed and stayed there for two days. I had reached a limit.

Arnold et al. (2020) call this experience camouflaging. I already felt different from other people. I just didn't understand why. Camouflaging is commonly known also as masking in the world of autism. Pearson et al. (2021) discuss the sheer energy that arises from masking as a response to stressors. Masking results in a disconnection between the real self and the perception of self, causing exhaustion and over-exertion, often unbeknownst to an undiagnosed person with autism. On reflection of my forty-four years, I have lost count of the many times I have masked to present the identity I thought would be acceptable. Up to the point of breaking. It is the snap of losing control that starts to bring the unconscious behaviour to the surface. Unfortunately, it is often too late and the masking has already resulted in a meltdown.

The idea of 'double consciousness' is also being used often in the world of autism now. This describes the need to evaluate behaviour based on the perception of the receiver. I remember as a young person I would imagine life as a game of chess. Life was really just a game and my actions were like moving a pawn in chess along an already decided board game. I questioned whether we were ever in control of our own destiny, but acting as a token instead. My actions were always in response to someone else. They still are in many ways. I may have a plan of how I would like to spend the day, but something happens. Life then becomes reactionary rather than taking action based on perceived messages. Again, this reactionary process is very draining and creates a feeling of just 'waiting'. Those people with a past history of trauma might understand here the feeling of just being on edge, being watched, and waiting until it is comfortable to act without caution.

In applying my yoga knowledge, I see this is an exacerbation of the nervous system, continually. The inner layer of the onion is on full alert, all the time. Applying my Ayurveda knowledge, I would suggest that the Vata, the elements of air and space, are way too high on the pendulum. In applying my youth work knowledge, we would look at this masking as the fight/flight mode in full swing. No wonder so many people with autism have dual diagnosis! It is exhausting to continually be on the lookout, to watch, process, respond according to the perceived expectations within the social environment, often also being overloaded by sensory stimulation.

The purpose of masking is to be able to associate in the world. Marged Goode, in her discussion with the Asperger's Victorian Group in 2021, suggested masking is ok, provided the participant does not become overloaded. This is a lovely way of accepting learned behaviour to function in a neurotypical society; however, it might still suggest there is something inherently flawed in the individual and there is something that remains unacceptable as a behavioural response for the general public.

Social media groups float the term alexithymia to explain their difficulties with identifying and processing emotions. In their research on social identity and autism, Pearson et al. (2020) suggest up to 50% of people diagnosed with autism have some form of alexithymia. To continue to mask or camouflage in social situations further confuses the identification of feelings, causing skills in emotional regulation and self-identification to be more difficult to achieve.

It is interesting to note according to Cage et al. (2020) the level of autistic identity and the relationship to camouflaging. They found that people who identify more strongly with autism are more likely to disclose that they are autistic, resulting not only in less stress, but also a stronger sense of self-identify and higher quality of life. The requirement to process emotions is supported to transpire according to the level of the individual and not based on a perception of societal demands. This behaviour also supports less stigma, and counteracts the medical model of autism as a deficit in something, an inherent flaw as opposed to a different way of seeing things.

The disclosure of autism may be a challenge. I had to read my environment. There were times as an adult when I just couldn't mask. It was just too difficult. As a teenager it was pretty obvious there was something wrong. I looked emaciated. As an adult, I still knew there was something a little left of centre but I looked fine; I was physically very fit, it was just that I didn't fit. How hard is it for people to understand when you don't even understand yourself?

Sometimes people with autism look just fine. They present so well that it is hard to believe in a diagnosis. Let's face it, I had enough trouble believing myself until I seriously looked into what autism really was. The diagnosis of autism requires that there is significant impairment. As autism is a spectrum, that impairment is going to look very different for different people.

This is where gaslighting starts to rear its ugly head. It wasn't until I was diagnosed with autism that I first heard the term gaslighting. I remember being so upset that my brothers and my mother had refused to believe my diagnosis, and that I had also copped abuse on top of it, that I turned to Facebook social media for support. Facebook groups, at the time of my diagnosis, were magnificent. Someone posted that I had been gaslighted. I had questioned my own sanity and diagnosis against the words of some ill-informed ignorance. When we first told my parents-in-law about our children and their diagnosis, the reason, they put forward, was the amount of technology we allowed them to use. The problem is we appear too normal. This makes autism become a hidden disability, and caused me further trauma, resulting in me having to just let go of the messages that I was deficient in some way. I was enough. I just had to learn to realise that.

As a female adult with a new diagnosis at the age of 43 I tried my diagnosis out on a few people around me. Some people were brilliant. Some people just accepted it and didn't talk any further about it. I really needed to talk though. I think, on reflection, it is really hard to understand the level of disability when the person presents so well. I look well. Plain and simple. I have multiple qualifications. I am a full-time mother. I run a full-time business. I have evolved in entrepreneurship. How on earth could I possibly have a disability that requires support? Aha! The art of masking at its best! Autism is a hidden disability.

Recently I became upset over a Facebook ad depicting yoga therapy for clients on the National Disability Insurance Scheme (NDIS). The advertisement showed a 'normal 'person with a person with Down syndrome. How do you achieve a visual representation of an invisible disability like autism? I really don't have the answers, but until the perceptions change, I know that I will need to continue to mask for some social contexts and that at the end of a day of masking I need to hide away and recover my energy. This is such a different way of responding to my life than reacting as an adult with borderline personality disorder.

Finally, finally, finally, after 43 years of searching, I can begin to let go of my perception of my social self, of how I am being perceived by others, and start to repair the damage that has been caused by rejecting the parts of myself that were deemed unsuitable, and to embrace my different way of thinking about things, developing a new perception of myself as a fully functional, non-deficient woman, who lives with autism.

For me, my ideal world right now is between the hours of 6.30 - 9.30pm. This is when my mask is removed; it's very similar to the feeling of taking off a bra at night. I can put on my pyjamas. For my last birthday my husband bought me an Oodie and it is thick and warm and heavy. I just love it. This goes on every night, giving me a gigantic hug. The kids go to bed and I can settle. I know there is much less chance of any surprises, of anything that requires me to mask, and all the thoughts I've been processing and psychological resources I've been depleting throughout the day can be recharged.

Chapter 10
Parenting With Autism - Recognising The Traits

My son told my yesterday on one of our drives that when I had meltdowns, before my diagnosis, I would come and seek him out and make him do stuff: vacuum, clean his room, take out the recycling etc. Parenting with autism is hard. Taking a relook at the diagnosis of autism, it becomes really clear there are issues with communication. Call these deficits if you will, but I am going to call them challenges.

My son talks about his flavour of the month. He becomes obsessed with five things and they rotate. For one month he is fully consumed by dinosaurs, then it becomes Lego, Warhammer, Pokémon and Star Wars. I get lost and I can't seem to keep up. He speaks a language I often can't follow. His passion can be expensive. I cannot tell you how much money he has saved up and spent on Warhammer or dinosaur figurines only to become obsessed with Lego the next day. I now understand what is happening. He has been so engrossed with the one subject matter that it has exhausted him.

My son is nearly thirteen and is newly diagnosed with autism. I didn't recognise it until after I was diagnosed. I have read a lot since my diagnosis and many of the stories are about parents of children who have autism who find out they, too, have it. For us it was the other way around. It explains so much!

My husband had this desire to move to the country. A few years earlier he had taken me on a horse-riding adventure and his dream was to have a long driveway up to the main house and a horse to run alongside his car as he drove home. He got his wish and we moved to the country. It was a long drive from the south-eastern suburbs to our home. Our little boy was three months old when we made the transition, with many trips there and back. He used to fall asleep to this one album of children's songs. Only this album. One day we didn't have it with us. My husband and I sang the songs. We knew it by heart by then. He settled and fell asleep. We were both amazed.

When he was two years old, my son discovered television. He loved it from the first moment he saw it. He gets addicted so easily to that set, to the exclusion of everything else. Our middle daughter was born at the time and I had visions of sitting in a particular rocking chair overlooking the paddocks feeding my newborn with my son by my side. Unfortunately, this new baby was super duper fussy. She would only feed when it was silent and we were on our own. So, for a worn-out mother, the television became the babysitter for when the baby was hungry. Not ideal, I know.

I would sit with my son and snuggle up to Iggle Piggle. I wasn't really into baby talk but he loved it! I would watch his head moving, almost involuntarily. I would watch him clicking his tongue. It was always very noisy sitting with him. When I mentioned what were obvious tics, my husband said he had also experienced tics and had grown out of them as an adult. My mother was also living with us for a short time and she was a maternal and child health nurse - surely, I had nothing to worry about. No one else had picked anything up except for me.

My son was also obsessed with Thomas the Tank Engine. Being the good parents we are, we went out and bought him loads of Thomas trains, complete with tracks and special track features. He didn't play with them. I would become angry and tell him to play with his tracks. When we had an adult friend come to stay, he would build tracks with him, but never on his own. Each train, however, was loved. At least two or three trains would be taken on every outing, never played with, just held and fiddled with. The wheels would be turned, the colours talked about, the names identified. He knew everything about those trains but never did he instigate play on his own.

The poor blossom started kindergarten. He did really well. I noticed him starting to complain about headaches, which became more and more frequent. I had also noticed his eyes beginning to water a lot. In my family, when I was growing up, unless we were bleeding or vomiting, we were pretty much dismissed. I told him to drink more water. I had suspected poor eyesight but I had taken him to two optometrists and both times the results had come back negative. His eyesight was deemed to be fine.

One day we took the train down to Melbourne to visit my in-laws. I had a pram and an absolutely miserable four year old. His eyes were red, he was sneezing, and he was just plain uncomfortable. I'd had enough. This was six months of battling this issue. When we arrived in Melbourne, I asked my father-in-law to take me straight to the doctors. This stoic little boy had two blood tests to rule out any allergies. The results: nada. Nothing. Negative. It wasn't until six months later when we realised what the problem was. His eyesight! The poor thing had really poor eyesight. He got glasses but the tics persisted.

When he was six my husband and I decided to move. This meant a change of primary school for my son. He was not happy. We ended up living in a caravan during the build and I trekked the forty-five-minute drive to and from his old school for the last term of the year. Over the summer he fretted. We had so many talks about the new school. He also developed a toilet fetish. We were using a builders' dunny that was out in the paddocks, about five metres from the caravan. Every night he would be restless, asking to go to the toilet up to 11pm at night. This was a challenge. I was used to going to bed by 10pm. My husband became angry. I became angry. The poor kid withdrew. It was the summer holidays and the days were hot. We decided to go on an overseas trip. My son's first comment was whether there would be a toilet on the plane. The penny dropped. This was an expression of anxiety and I had completely misread the situation.

So now I knew what I was dealing with, as a mother I could act. We coached him and encouraged him. I thought things were going pretty well. I had given him a placebo lolly as a magic bladder controller for a few weeks and we had noticed a difference. I was so proud of him, and myself. One day his teacher came up to me and asked if my son had a bladder problem. She told me every half hour he had to go to the bathroom and it was interfering with his work. Damn.

Fast forward a few years to Grade Four. My son is an avid reader. He just devours books. I had been a hands-on mum as much as I could handle and we had read together most mornings before school. One day in the classroom the teacher told him to put away his books in his special book box. I had no idea my son was so disengaged in the classroom he would hide books all around the room. The teacher's response was not to tell me, but to use a book box for him to store his books. An interesting flip on having to get a kid to stop reading, as opposed to encouraging reading.

For his fifth year of school my husband and I made the decision to make another change for our son. His youngest sister was due to start school the next year and we thought a bigger school might be a better fit. One evening we sat the children down and told them they would be starting a new school term four of that year. Whew, was he upset. For those two weeks I coached, I consoled, and my son slept beside my bed. I now recognise a sign of anxiety caused by, at that stage, undiagnosed autism.

He did really well at this new school. He found a group of friends and things were looking up. I was so pleased for him. Sometimes I would become frustrated with him, like when he would just disappear, or when he would talk about the same thing over and over, but we were going along well. I was aware there were definite likes and dislikes which I assumed were part of his personality. He didn't excel at sport. Big deal, I thought. Hence my surprise when he asked me to take him to Auskick. I was literally blown away. His reason for Auskick was to learn skills. Ok, I got up Sunday mornings like other parents for the frosty 9am beginnings. When I asked him if he wanted to continue with football and join a club the response was a blanket no. His purpose had been achieved in simply learning skills.

I run my own business and one of the luxuries of this is being able to navigate my working hours around the children. For my son's Grade Five camp I put my hand up to attend. Yup, me who has structure and routine would be, for the next three days at least, immersed in the school structure. I watched and observed. One of the evening events was a music quiz. The music was LOUD. Super Duper Loud! I watched my son put his head down on the table and block his ears. Here comes Mumma Bear. I swooped in and took him and a few other kids outside. The teachers made no response. I thought he was just being a bit of a sook. I had no idea at that stage the pain of sensory overload on his hearing. If I didn't know, how on earth could the teachers know?

Warhammer became one of his main interests. As a parent, I struggle with the name. Hey, I also struggle with the name Star Wars. I saw, though, that his interest and the game itself involved computers, art and role playing. Bingo! Just what this kid needed. So, we started down the Warhammer path. He had this vision of a Warhammer group at school. He prepared a presentation for his principal and with a little guidance from his teacher he was successful in starting the first lunchtime club.

Bang. Covid. Grade Six. Such expectations. School camp: cancelled. Warhammer club: cancelled. Social interaction: cancelled. Needless to say, one of the positives for him was the amount of time spent on technology as a result of home schooling but it also caused friction between us and I had to police it. He would often talk with nostalgia about all the things he was meant to do and wasn't able to do. I get it. It was unfair. Even more importantly though, it was out of routine and the set structure that he had prepared himself for.

The transition between primary and high school is difficult for lots of people. I was beginning to read my son. I saw the transition and the unknown for him was causing lots of anxiety. I pulled in my high school teacher husband to intervene. One of the greatest fears was the bus. Again, the dreaded school bus - I knew all too well the inability to be flexible when it came to the school bus. He was also separated from his primary school peer group. On reflection, one of the biggest things I would change for him is sticking my nose in and asking for him to be in the same class as his primary school mates. Transition for kids on the spectrum is just plain hard.

Around mid-April we had visited a paediatrician for all of our children. My research on autism had identified traits and I had concerns. Autism characteristics include differences in communication and social interaction. My son had this wonderful half smile that he would give. His eye contact was sporadic. Toe walking and a body position that was almost like he was going to trip was common. What more evidence did I really need here? The tics that he had as a child were still persistent. His preferred activity was to be on his own reading or, if he was allowed to, playing computer games, oblivious to his surroundings.

Our communication was often fraught with misunderstandings. He would become flustered when talking with me. His breath became laboured and shoulders tense. Often, he would give up and I would become frustrated. My frustration presents as anger. Then the merry go round begins and it is even harder for him to get a word out. So, I am learning. He is learning. I am learning that he is very very literal. If I say bring an umbrella he will walk with an umbrella even if it isn't raining. If I speak, I need to make sure that I am understood. There is a lot of confusion and a lot of misunderstandings that get us both frustrated and, thank goodness, end up in lots of hugs. The transition from primary school to high school is difficult for mothers. Suddenly we lose track of what is happening. I am experiencing this and I need to be on my toes because things like free dress day at school just get lost in his translation, and I don't want him to be the only kid in uniform at school ever again!

Every night for two years I was a confidante. My experience as a youth worker and my one personal experience had taught my some pretty good counselling skills. I also had my autism ability to read a situation to back me up. Every night I would tuck my girl into bed and we would debrief. Sometimes I was exhausted by it. Sometimes I just wished she would tell Daddy because I felt at a loss. I didn't want to see her in pain, but she chose to confide in me, and as a mother I would support her until the day the cows came home.

Being a girl can be tough. Let's face it. Being a girl with autism presents a different challenge, particularly when it comes to friendships. It took until Grade Three for my girl to find a friend. She loved this friend and we could see the feeling was mutual. A feature of autism is an all-consuming approach to friendship. One on one, this works just fine. To 'read 'a friend there is a lot of unconscious thought put into the relationship but it is only for one person. Add a third person into the blend and you have issues. Now it becomes harder to be able to 'read 'the behaviours of the third person and to understand what is happening with the different dynamics of the relationships.

I was amazed by how insightful my girl was. She watched. She could relay to me every little action and behaviour of the third friend, even down to the fine detail of swinging a bracelet. Wow; that takes a lot of energy.

So, night after night we would debrief and I would listen to her analyse every move and behaviour that was happening in class. She just couldn't understand it and I could see she was in a lot of pain. A year before she had tried to develop a relationship with two girls and was the odd wheel out. In her words, one of the mothers had told the girls not to play with my girl because she was too bossy. I had no idea how to console her about this and I am still not sure if it was her interpretation or if it was true.

Nonetheless, she was upset. Really upset. With real tears every night. I put it down to part of growing up, because girls can be bitchy. I had experienced enough of this when I was growing up. Patiently I would listen and try and help her pull things apart to make sense of it all.

Around this time, she started leaving me little notes in the doorway. I thought it was cute. I started to write back. She would tell me little things through her words. How she felt. What I needed to do. What she needed to do. After a month or so I asked her if we could keep these notes and start to write in a little diary. A firm no was what I got. The routine was to write on scrap bits of paper and leave the notes in the doorway. Strategy! I went with her and we bought a Harry Potter book. Aha! Now we had somewhere to keep all these notes and her bedroom and mine became less cluttered with little bits of scrap paper everywhere. It was also a really good way to keep track of how she was doing and I thought it would make a great diary for her to reflect on later in life.

For the last year we have been writing every night in this diary. If I miss a night, she tells me off, in the diary. If I use a different pen, if I put it back in a different spot, she tells me off in her diary. This diary is telling me so so much about my girl.

Routine and structure and organisation are her strengths. She is very analytical and a very good people watcher. She is also extremely sensitive and like her brother will read for hours on end. I believe she is up to her ninth time of reading the full Harry Potter series through. It took great effort to get her interested in a different series.

Unlike her brother, she is extremely organised. Everything has its place and it needs to be in that place. When I walk into her room, I just see chaos, but she knows where everything is and has her little ways. For sleep she needs her blue blanket and her special eye pillow. Anything Harry Potter is acceptable and she has collected a vast display of Harry Potter memorabilia.

When she shuts down though, she is very different from her brother. She just cannot communicate. She can grunt. I can see her flinch. Sometimes she would stay like this for hours. I found it really frustrating because I couldn't seem to work out what the switch was. She would just go into one of her moods and it took her ages to come out of it. She is also stubborn, which can be a positive thing but it was hard to deal with.

Remember my vision of her as a baby? Me, sitting in a particular chair, with my son next to me, looking out at the paddocks and feeding my little girl. Nope. Right from the beginning she had her own agenda. She would not attach to feed unless it was just her and me. No stimulation. No brother. No tv. Just the two of us.

Meal times were a disaster. I absolutely dreaded feeding her as a baby. She would just point-blank refuse and I would end up tearing my hair out. At that time, I was pretty strung out with two children and managing a lot of my overload with alcohol. I had no idea I was dealing with autism for myself as well, so as soon as it got to around 3-4pm I would start the road of self-medication. Often my husband would need to take over feeding my girl solids when he came home from work. I found it just too overwhelming.

There were certain textures she just wouldn't eat. Now I have zero tolerance for this, as does my husband. Neither of us have experienced allergies or fussy eaters and we expect the kids to eat what we are providing them. Why she wouldn't eat rice? I had no idea. I honestly thought she was just being a brat. We began to notice when the texture was smooth, she would struggle to swallow. Sometimes we would just sit there for an hour saying to her just swallow the damn food. We would take the food away and then reserve it to her for the next meal. Nope. She would refuse to budge. It was not going to be eaten.

Maybe because she was the middle child, my girl was overlooked. She met all her developmental milestones. Yes, she was sometimes fussy, but aren't all kids at some stage? I just thought she was my fussy one. I had no clue whatsoever when she was younger that there might be more to my girl than meets the eye.

Until middle primary school. Then she started to become a little obsessive in her behaviour and her communication traits became apparent. She would write to me about her little habits. Sometimes it was having to touch something. Sometimes it was flexing her elbows. She called them her annoying little habits and they appeared to really bother her. Her behaviours of autism were so subtle I nearly missed them. It was only through learning about myself that I started to question the hours I was spending every week debriefing with her and coaching her need to analyse her friend's behaviours.

It wasn't until she reached Grade Five that I became really convinced she had autism. I have never interfered with my children's grade allocation; however, her distress about the friendship situation was increasing and I asked her classroom teacher to separate her from some of her peers. This did not go down well with her, as you may imagine. I spent weeks coaching her on what the classroom would look like the next year. Most of the coaching would happen in the evenings, just before bed, when she was overloaded and I was exhausted. Still, I loved her and she needed support.

The week before school began she was in tears most nights. When school started, I spent many evenings with her literally planning out what to say. We would rehearse in the car so she had some sentence starters. We did this naturally. Marged Goode in her presentation with Asperger's Victoria identified some of the behaviours associated with masking. My girl and I were practising social skills. We had pre-scripted what she was going to say and how she was going to act. My girl was obsessed with *Fuller House* and would replay episode after episode learning social skills. She was needing support to socialise and understand her role in social situations.

My husband and I would literally coach her, at meal times, on how to answer questions in class. We told her to put her hand up to answer every second question, not every question. For a girl with autism this was nonsensical. If the teacher asks a question and you know the answer, you put your hand up. She was noticing, however, the response of her classmates, which was confusing her - they saw her as a goody two shoes. All of this is behind the scenes work. If I had not been identified as having autism, I would still be consoling her and being frustrated by her meltdowns and shutdowns.

Recently my girl joined a gym class. I finally got it together to book both my girls into gym. It had to be a particular gym that my girl had previously visited with the school; any suggestion at all to join a different gym was met with an instant shutdown. Sometimes you just choose the battles you need to fight, so I let go of trying to help her with adaptation and was pleased that she was doing something active and that she really enjoyed her gym.

Then she slipped and broke her arm. My kids cry. If there is the slightest little bump or scrape it's a catastrophe, so when I got a call that she had hurt her arm, I dismissed it. I had things to do and I drove home with her. She had gone into a closed meltdown and wouldn't let me near her. I used the television as a soother for her. An hour later I had a look. Crap. It was hot, hard and swollen to buggery. This arm was broken. My husband took her to the hospital and it was confirmed. Broken.

All good. We coped with this and made our adjustments. In fact, she coped really well with some of the changes we had to make, and I was able to intercede in most of the meltdowns - with one exception. On the day of review, we waited an hour and half at the hospital. I was so paranoid I arrived 45 minutes early, unintentionally. I was told the doctors were seeing patients by order of arrival so we decided to wait. People with autism are known to take things literally. We counted down the patients and we were next. This wasn't too bad. Except we weren't next. Patient after patient was seen. Every so often a doctor would hold the door open longer than usual and the beep was sending my sensory overload insane. I think I may have actually groaned at one stage.

At the X-ray session my girl was told she would have another cast. Or maybe it was at Emergency on the night she broke it. Anyway, we were talking about colours and designs. When she was seen by the doctor, he told her there was no cast change required. In fact, he told her that if he did change the cast there would be more chance of disturbing the healing that had taken place to date. I saw her face fall.

This was a girl who had meticulously planned who was going to write on the cast and where. She had even considered writing everyone's names in order so it was acceptable to her. She had told all her classmates they could write on the cast. The current one was heavy and was covered by a bandage held in a sling, so any signing was impossible. Hello meltdown.

It took two hours for her to come out of it. She shut down. She snapped. She just retreated inside. Eventually she was able to identify, with my encouragement, her disappointment. It was the second last day of term the next day and I told her she could have the day off if she chose. The waiting and change of circumstances had exhausted us all. I picked up a Texta and wrote my name through the bandage and tucked her into bed.

The next morning, the meltdown resurfaced. She spilt milk on her clothes. This was the straw that broke the camel's back, and she changed back into her pyjamas. To her credit she told me that if something happened at school today, she was already overloaded and wouldn't be able to handle it. Autism is so strong for her. She had a vision. To ask her to shift her vision is very very difficult. It required a cognitive restructure of her script and the pre-conceived responses of her peers, and she just didn't have the capabilities to handle it. So she stayed home with me, and I learned a valuable lesson: don't arrive early to appointments!

In the midst of my son starting kindergarten for the first time, my baby was born. I had experienced both an emergency Caesar and a natural birth and I was pushing for another natural birth. This baby, however, had her own ideas. She twisted into transverse position. So, I did yoga poses. I did chiropractic therapy. I did Chinese medicine. Nope. She swung back the other way into breech. I fought for her to come when she chose and pushed back against the recommendation for induced labour. Nope. She decided she wanted to hang on well past her due date. My baby always had her own way of doing things.

When she was born, she was great. My easiest baby ever! She was so quiet. She was so agreeable. I could take her anywhere at any time and she just accepted it. My baby was just lovely. I have fond memories of my son at kinder with my girl playing alongside him. My baby would sit in the pram happily waiting whilst I chopped the fruits for kinder snack. This year was my highlight of motherhood.

My baby met all the developmental milestones. I had no reason to question anything, but I found being a mother to her was beginning to get interesting. She most definitely had her own ideas. She would go first in everything. She rushed to open a door before me, meaning that I would be waiting while she struggled to open it. As an already overloaded mother with sensory and emotional dysregulation I was triggered. The only problem was, I had no idea what was happening.

I was also dry by this stage. I had not touched one drop of alcohol since finding out I was pregnant with my baby and to this day, I never have and never will. My autistic all or nothingness would not allow even one drop of alcohol to pass my lips and I knew this was our last child, so any drinking had to stop.

My baby was challenging. She would just lose it. She would snap. Her attitude was sometimes so lovely and then out of the blue she would change and become defiant. She yelled at the other kids. She spoke with aggression. I was told it was just developmental and she would grow out of it. So, I waited.

When she was in kindergarten my husband asked me to get her hearing checked. No way. My mother was trained as a child health nurse and we would sit across from her at the table and whisper. She always responded. It turned out her hearing was very low and she needed grommets to unblock the wax from her ears. I was told after this I would have a better-behaved child. Well, the grommets went in, but the behaviour remained unchanged. I was being pushed to my limits and started asking for help. The only issue was, I wasn't really sure what I was asking for, and I had enough of my own mental health issues to deal with.

We went in for a second lot of grommets when she started primary school. My husband at this stage was concerned with her ability to read and was starting to question whether she might have dyslexia. I had approached the kindergarten teacher on his behalf with the concerns, and they were dismissed, with the reasoning that she was too social. In her first year of primary school again I approached the teacher, midyear, again to be dismissed. By term three however I requested my baby repeat the year and the teacher conceded. She repeated the school year.

I was told that my baby was an angel in school. She was so well behaved. She demonstrated compassion and was responsive to her peers. I didn't experience this. As soon as she got into the car after school, I had an aggressive little girl. She would scowl. She grunted. She snapped all of our heads off if we looked sideways. This was exhausting and I was always so disappointed, having looked forward to seeing the kids after school. My energy was draining.

We went in for the third lot of grommets. I hoped against hope there would be a change in behaviour and the little girl that was so pleasant in school would be the little girl I would see at home. Nope. We took her in for eye testing, knowing that my son's eyesight was very limited. Surprise - she also had poor eyesight, and needed strong glasses. Ok, this had to be the reason she was reading backwards and not retaining her words. It had to be the reason every time I tried to read with her it ended up in frustration. We had found our answer! Fancy trying to get a little person to read when they can't hear properly and they can't see the words clearly.

The only thing was that it didn't work. The behaviour at home remained the same, if not worse. Time after time the teachers said she was an angel at school. I had a girl who would become easily frustrated the moment she got in the car with me, and I was tired.

Covid came, and with it came lockdown. This meant her whole routine was tipped upside down and I had the joys of home-schooling. We got some baby ducklings and hand reared them. I have memories of her sitting online with her computer, little yellow duckling in hand. My baby loves animals! School had routine. I struggle with routine. We started to flounder. I was also trying to support my other two children and a husband, who were all at home. Her aggression was increasing.

My solution was to map out each day with a timetable. My goodness, it worked! She took to it like a duck to water. She knew what to do. She would keep us all in check if we were late or if we strayed past the time. This child thrived on routine.

Time and again I would ask for help when she was younger. I hit rock bottom and told the nurse at the hospital that I was struggling with the aggression. It was quick to start up and quick to dissipate. It was ignored. I told my husband. Developmental and personality, I was told. He told his counsellor. Again, the same response. I was advised to practise restorative justice for behavioural management at home with her but I wasn't convinced.

She was a remarkable child, one on one. So loving and caring. She also demonstrated compassion. She had the innate ability to read when someone was in pain and was there straight away to offer comfort, even to her siblings. She showed so much love and care to our puppy. Such an animal lover was she that any sign of hurt or neglect towards animals on television affected her for days on end.

For restorative justice though, the ability to demonstrate remorse and reflect on the circumstances was required. This I could not see. I would punish her - take things away, ban her from things she liked, or offer her rewards. Really, she didn't seem to care. It was almost like she had disassociated from whatever was happening and she couldn't connect the dots. I was exhausted. I left it to my husband to manage her.

He tried the best he knew how. He tried to reason with her. I stood back and observed. He would imitate her behaviour and ask her to respond. She was so good at providing all the correct responses that were expected of her. I doubted her sincerity and her ability to understand what was happening. In all of our discussions the terms 'developmental stage 'and 'personality 'were discussed. I felt blocked.

By the time I had my autistic breakdown I was done. As far as I could see, there was no growing out of the aggression and it was becoming worse. Sometimes she would just look at me and grin with an almost eerie smile on her face. It was completely disconnected from what was happening. She would be on the floor throwing a tantrum but it was kind of different from the stereotypical version of a tantrum. She would close off and then suddenly come back to us. She would write me little letters and throw them at me, spelling words the best she could. I would hear her in her room yelling 'help me', and 'I don't understand'. I was at a loss.

Autism. I saw it. I flagged up to my husband. Yes, so far, my presentation on the other two children had him concede that they both might have autism. As to my baby, he remained unconvinced, still insisting it was developmental, personality and possibly dyslexia. A mumma knows. I had no tools and I was tired. I fought against this one and eventually he agreed to have her tested along with the other two children.

By this stage I had already understood her inability to reason. I saw her frustration that her older siblings wouldn't play with her the way she wanted them to play. I saw how unsettled she was at night and I was beginning to see similar friendship patterns occur that had crippled my daughter.

Finally, finally, finally she had a teacher who had also observed some behaviours of autism in my baby. Finally, I was not the only person who didn't believe that my baby was just going through a developmental stage or that her behaviour was just part of her personality. The Jekyll and Hyde transformation was obvious. She played a role and she played it well when things were structured and clear for her. When the boundaries become blurred, she flounders. Enter what looks like aggression, as she fights to manage her anxiety.

The last lockdown in Covid was the hardest yet. Her expectations once again had changed. I could not do anything with her. Every single activity would result in her stomping off and yelling. We went for a drive to calm her, and me. We played eye spy in the car and stopped at a country park. All of us came along and it was a family adventure. Even the dog came! We had fun. My son drew out dinosaur footprints in the bark, a sign of his latest obsession. She came along and filled them in. Wait. Stop. What? Suddenly the tide turned again. He was upset. She became disagreeable and inconsolable. What the hell had just happened?

We drove home. My son was distraught but not saying anything. I saw his internalised meltdown. My baby on edge. Me, just driving. Things had to change.

I rang the school and asked for my baby to be able to attend. They agreed. She loved it. She was back in her routine and structure and she did what was expected of her. We saw a changed child. Classic autism.

Chapter 11
Diagnosing Childhood Autism & Early Intervention

To have a formal diagnosis for my children, I had to have two forms of evidence, and both of these had to be further verified by the paediatrician to confirm that the children did have autism. This sounds simple. It is not. Firstly, one of the forms of evidence had to be from a psychologist who had performed an assessment known as the Autistic Diagnostic Observation Schedule (ADOS). Finding a psychologist that was available without a huge long waiting list was a marathon effort.

The second form of evidence could be from either a speech therapist or an occupational therapist. Again, sounds simple. Just choose one. I had no idea though that speech therapists did anything other than work with children with lisps. I thought occupational therapists were for old people to keep them in their homes or for people in rehabilitation who had broken an arm or something.

Here came a huge learning curve. Speech therapists can help children with social skills. Knowing that people with autism have differences in social communication, this made sense to me. I chose this option. All the waiting lists were full. I had three children who all required assessments. I was looking at a ten-month waiting period at least, and that was considered to be a short wait. Not for me. I rang therapists in Melbourne and then hit New South Wales. My yellow book was full of names, charges, phone numbers and referrals made left right and centre. I found someone and was making appointments, and then I discovered something else.

During this time, I had been struggling to cope with the multitude of demands. I was burning out fast and felt like I had the responsibility of all of these children on my shoulders. I was also suffering with mother guilt that I had given them a curse of autism. I had struggled so much in my life and the thought of my beloved children experiencing any of the pain I had experienced filled me with absolute horror.

I had an appointment with a National Disability Insurance Scheme (NDIS) to review my plan given I now had a new diagnosis that included autism. This reviewer listened and asked me about whether I'd had assessments with an occupational therapist (OT). She was pretty clear that an OT assessment would provide advice on day to day living and this concept that was really new to me called executive functioning.

Executive functioning skills help to organise thoughts and are essential for mental processing. When there is a difference in executive functioning skills it can be difficult to manage everyday life. Take for example ordering a school lunch for the kids via the new online system. That is just a nightmare. The multitude of emails and posts that come out from school is overwhelming and most of the time I just delete them. It's not that I don't care, it is just too much to process. I much preferred the old-fashioned newsletters and handwritten permission notes from old times.

So, I learned from the NDIS review that unless there were specific areas that were identified as requiring support, it was very hard to make plans for supports. I also learned the value of reports from professionals in helping to access supports. OTs can offer sensory processing assessments as well. So that was where I decided to head with the children for their diagnostic reports.

Now came the ring around for OTs. Waiting lists again were huge and a lot of therapists had even closed their books. Again, I started researching Melbourne and as far as NSW. I meticulously recorded the details of therapists, waiting lists, fees and phone numbers in my yellow book. By this stage I was a walking directory of all the paediatricians, speech therapists, psychologists and occupational therapists from Victoria and New South Wales.

I also learned the art of asking to be placed on cancellation lists. Bingo. Within a month I had the first assessment booked for my child. The OT did a terrific job! I read the report we received a week later and it was excellent. The therapists had understood my child completely within that time period and we had concrete recommendations on how to support him. I was impressed, and I am a fussy client.

The other two children were also assessed within a month. Cancellation lists are gold and I would highly recommend anyone undergoing a diagnostic process to use that golden phrase 'please place me on your cancellation list'. Now I had an issue. I had three excellent reports on sensory processing with a clear picture of autism being revealed, but all the three children were different. One had sensory seeking behaviour and the other two had sensory avoidant behaviour; and then there was also myself to deal with as well. How on earth do I manage all of this and a husband who is still frantically trying to keep up with all of this whilst also holding down a full-time job and working hard to support a wife who it has been revealed is dependent on him to act as her carer?

It was pretty obvious to me that my children would be diagnosed with autism. I presented the evidence and sold it well to my husband, who agreed to pursue a diagnosis. The paediatrician also validated my observations, but would a psychologist be able to see what I saw when I wasn't in the room with the children? Would they assess the children as level 1 or level 2? If the children came back as level 1 then it would be very difficult to get funding to access support services and we would seriously need to consider how we would manage the children's additional needs. If the children were assessed as level 2, as I was, then there would be an automatic acceptance of the need for funded supports. What if only one child was diagnosed as level 1 and the other two children were diagnosed as level 2? Would this cause disagreement amongst them? It was a game of trust in the specialists, because essentially, they have your fate in their hands.

I am a good researcher. It is what I do. I have been researching ways to be healthy for most of my life. I am also very persistent. I have had to be because for most of my teenage years onwards I only had myself to rely on. So I found two psychologists: one for my baby, about whom I had additional concerns about dyslexia and ADHD, and a local therapist for my son and my girl. This is a lot of trust to place in a therapist. It is also expensive. My nerves were on edge. In the end, both therapists saw, independently from my observations, what I had assessed. All three of my children had level 2 autism.

My next step was to connect the children with service providers. This is not easy. Again, waiting lists are huge and despite autism being considered a spectrum, with individual traits being reflective of the individualised nature of the manifestation of autism, there is a generalised treatment program - OTs, speech therapy and counselling. The waiting lists! They are huge! Services are so stretched they close their books. In the meantime, every piece of research I come across screams at me early intervention. I was desperate to get my kids into services so history wouldn't repeat my pain; but how?

To help us navigate the world of service provision my children had also been issued with a support coordinator to access services, help them with their goals for living independently and growing and developing. One thing I don't understand is how this person will differ from what I do right now?

One of the biggest challenges is children. To work with children is a specialised area. To find therapists that work with children is one thing, but to find therapists that are available is another aspect altogether. I found an excellent therapist for my baby. She was so good! Ok, one down, two to go.

Now consider this dilemma. How important is it for the therapist to match the needs of the child? Sometimes we click, sometimes we don't. I had experienced many therapists myself in the past. One, who I paid highly at the time, fell asleep on me - twice. Another asked me if I had taken drugs and then proceeded to disclose to me drugs she had taken with her son. What?? So not only was I on the lookout for therapists for both my remaining children, but also therapists who would be a suitable fit for them to work with. I struggled with this, as I witnessed a few therapists who just didn't seem like a good fit. Was it better to keep the child in therapy knowing they would find engagement difficult, or stop the therapy altogether and wait for a good fit? After many discussions, ear bashing my husband, we agreed on the latter. For my girl we are still searching for the right therapist but for my son the gamble paid off and he has recently engaged with an excellent therapist that he not only agrees to see but is happy to see. This, I know, will definitely help to develop a therapeutic relationship for him.

The OT and speech therapists - where am I up to with them? Well, we continue to be on waiting lists. If I am lucky, maybe next year we will get a place. One of the challenges with services is not only obtaining diagnostic assessments, but also the availability of ongoing sessions. There is such a high demand, with already overly stretched resources, and I am playing a game of catch up as a late diagnosed mother suddenly presented with three children with autism.

Chapter 12
Strategies for Our Parenting

What really scares me is when I don't cope. I read reports that people with autism are more likely to experience dual diagnosis as a result of their difficulties in interacting with mainstream society. My diagnosis is a huge alphabet of acronyms. Not only am I bound with mum guilt for passing on the autism trait, but now I have to manage the possibility that my parenting style may lead to further disabilities in mental health issues for my children. Dissanayake et al. (2019) discuss the level of autistic traits and the reduced outcomes of healthy development in children. My autism is very well hidden after years of practise but it is definitely on the mid to high scale. Does this mean I won't be able to parent well? Not on my watch it doesn't! To compound things further, Dissanayake et al. (2019) also highlight that those difficulties in parenting can lead to reduced self-esteem in children and result in mental difficulties. So not only do I have to access support services for my children now, I also have to act as a responsible and emotionally available parent at all times, and somehow swallow my autistic traits that cause conflict, in order to raise emotionally resilient children. It was too much. I faltered.

I started to research parenting support programs for parents of children who had autism. This proved to be even more difficult than finding therapists for the three children. I contacted help lines that specialised in autism. I contacted local services. Most of the providers had support sessions down in the Melbourne area or were run online. This didn't suit me. I hate online support groups. I had already been traumatised by my experiences with the DBT groups and thanks in part to Covid a lot of the support had moved to online or was on fairly permanent pause a year later.

Really, apart from accessing online classes and sessions in autism I could not find support services to help families with newly diagnosed children learn how to manage autism. Again, I turned to social media in the form of Facebook and here I learned that I was not the only one who was struggling for support. There is a process parents move through on learning the diagnosis. One is relief. Their observations are finally validated and there is a reason for what has been happening. There is also a name for it, and in that moment, you join a tribe. Then there is grief. What you had hoped will be different. After receiving a diagnosis, the next step is action. Always action; the time for processing is never readily available, time to sit and actually reflect on what it means and how it is going to look. It just becomes a fight to try and navigate this new world and be an advocate for the children.

I saw this coming. I panicked and asked my husband if we could sell the Retreat. Suddenly everything I had hoped and lived for was different. I now had three children to care for and I was buggered if I was going to mess that up. I had a picture of what my weeks would now look like. We were on our own as a family, with no help from any extended family members, and what I was foreseeing was appointments for each child at least once a week. Alongside my own appointments this was going to equate to at least five appointments per week, which translates to approximately ten hours by the time I travel in and out. I was also studying full-time, teaching, and trying to run a business properly. Do the figures. As a school mum my work hours were already between the 9-3pm zone. Suddenly I had to cram everything in to 20 hours a week. It felt too heavy.

Is there the possibility that parents with autism who have children with autism are more attuned to their needs? According to Dissanayake et al. (2019), parents who are on the spectrum may experience increased difficulties in responding to their children's emotional needs and offering behavioural support based on role modelling and communication efficiency. In our home we have found this to be inaccurate. There is an innate strength in my ability to observe all the children and to recognise what is happening for them at a particular time.

Sometimes this is a strength and I can deflect a meltdown and provide proper support and guidance. When I am overloaded, I can see what is happening, almost like a bird's eye view of a land laid out before me, and bring in my husband to help with the diffusion. When I am heightened, however, it is a different story.

In this I would agree wholeheartedly with Dissanayake et al.'s (2019) reports that parents on the spectrum may have trouble controlling their own emotional needs against the needs of the children. When I am in sensory overload, or as we now say in our home, the yellow to red zone, I become unreasonable. I cannot hear properly. I have watched my own behaviour. I squint and move further forward to hear. It is very difficult to block things out and concentrate on what is being presented before me. This then dissipates any ability I might have to advocate for my child's needs. One of our biggest concerns is the availability of support that is accessible to help during this period.

We are now a family of five with four of us being diagnosed with autism level 2, amongst other diagnoses. I have the ability to be able to 'read' my children and sense when they are moving towards a meltdown response. Often, I need to direct my husband to this. He doesn't appear to have the same capability to be able to recognise when a situation has blown up, either in an outward display of a meltdown or in an internalised presentation of what constitutes a meltdown.

This is hard for both of us. Sometimes I become resentful that I have to manage all of our behaviours, and he can sense my frustration. I am sure there are times when he just becomes overwhelmed himself; however, we all have a diagnosis that might perhaps in some way be a presentable response to the situation, and he is expected just to keep on keeping on without the same leniency or opportunity to process afforded to him.

Some of the strategies we have put in place so far are for sensory reducing or sensory seeking. We have one child who is sensory seeking, I am a combination of both and my oldest two children are both sensory avoidant. This means only one of the children is looking for constant stimulation whilst the other two are trying to retreat. Me, well, I also have attention deficit disorder along with other labels so I am just a fish in a pond of labels and I am ok with that. Sometimes I want stimulation, sometimes I can't stand it.

For example, right now I am writing whilst listening to meditation music. Other times when I write I need silence. Sometimes I can't look at a computer screen. It is this inconsistency which can drive my husband sometimes to despair as he tries to work out what to do in each situation, as if it was predictable from the one before. Unfortunately, my autism does not present like that.

By now all three children had been in for their diagnostic assessments and they all had a diagnosis of autism level 2, and my baby had a form of dyslexia but not ADHD. I sat on the couch with the kids one day and started looking at autism stores for sensory regulation. I saw these behaviour charts. This was similar to what I had learned in my study days as a youth worker. Righto. I had a strategy for the first time. I sat with the girls and we made time out charts. They chose each activity and the pictures to match. They chose the colour schemes and the fonts. I pulled out my feelings cards and we selected six feelings. I made reward charts and they chose their own tokens. I selected a behaviour regulation chart with visual representations for the different zones of blue, green, yellow and red. I printed them out and laminated them.

My gosh, it worked. I had a strategy. The pieces of the puzzle were starting to fit. Slowly we are growing. One of our other most effective tools is the reward chart. This is golden. The kids all have their own goals and ten rewards equals time on the devices. We haven't quite reached the 'I feel' charts but we do talk in a new language. Emotional dysregulation and 'I'm in the yellow zone 'are now part of our everyday language.

The desperation I was feeling for someone to help is not as strong as it was and a lot of my actions are supported by the new educational psychologist we have for my baby. Recently she told me it is too much to expect my baby to know how to self-regulate when she is in the yellow/red zones and she really does need guidance to help reduce the heightened state. Instead of needing to run away I am now more able to help her, and my husband is understanding her inability to reason. Slowly, slowly, we are learning how to be parents of children diagnosed with autism level 2, emotional dysregulation and dyslexia. It is a journey we are still discovering.

I often ask the kids what zone they are in. Finally, the reward chart was something tangible my baby responded to. My girl in a meltdown one day slammed a sad face on the feelings poster. My husband during a discussion told me he was moving into the yellow zone. We took a pause before resuming the conversation.

I bought whiteboards. We put one in each of the children's rooms and a huge one in the family area. I offloaded all of my list onto the big board. It worked. I wrote down times of things we do and when. It worked. At the moment it is still working. Sometimes I have enough and it is hard to keep going, but the kids and the parents are adapting to the new language.

Whiteboards, markers, colours, erasers. These are four words that have made a profound difference to our day to day living. It gets stuff out of my head. It helps the kids learn to read and write, particularly my baby with her dyslexia. Part of letting go of micro managing is allowing the kids to do what we need them to do in their own time. It may seem logical to others but for me it wasn't. It was outside the rule book. We are all learning. Colours as well are great for us to see what is important and who it relates to. My baby is highly visual and this is helping her sensory processing. Part of the whiteboard is also a pin board which is great for school notices and the like. I can't forget when it is in my face and this helps with executive functioning. I also refuse to rub out the cute little bird one of the kids drew on the side.

Against all my better judgement we put the children on melatonin, following the paediatrician's advice. We thought it was just normal that the children bounced up and down for a couple of hours before they settled. Most families talk about how difficult it is to get their children to sleep and given the children slept mostly through the night we weren't concerned. What we were unaware of was the anxiety the children faced before going to sleep. The melatonin made such a difference. The children started to settle well and the bouncing stopped. We definitely noticed they had an easier time settling at night.

We have a huge tub of fidget toys. These are great. I hate some of the ones that feel tight, but my baby loves them. My son loves the big chucky ones. My girl likes the creative ones like make your own slime and then the cool feeling between her hands. She also likes the structure of the pop it plastic fidget toys and I do believe she is in some kind of competition to get the most fidget toys amongst her friendship group. We keep these toys in a tub so we are all clear on where they go and I don't get overloaded by so many little (and big) things around the house.

Socks and shoes can be a nightmare. I had no idea before we had our autism diagnosis what the girls were actually talking about. They are both stimulated by the feeling of the sewed line at the top of the toes. Me and my son, we couldn't care less. So, we invested in some sensory socks without that line. They, too, are thrown into a big tub and they are all white to help reduce the panic that was coming when I would call out,' Five minutes before we are going! 'This would send my baby into a sock and shoe meltdown! We still haven't quite got to the shoes yet, but we are nailing the sock issue.

Where would we be without the BIG visual timer? This is also a godsend. It helps us all keep track of time. We set it and the amount of time we are wanting will be in red. This reduces as time goes by ending with a big ring. The only issue is I can't stand the tick and it can be ineffective when the kids have headphones on.

Noise cancelling headphones work for my baby. She has a headset that she just loves. This is perfect for when she needs her own personal time out. She also really loves music and she can listen away to her heart's content to her Descendants Disney songs! Me, I find the noise cancelling scary. I hear a buzz. It is too quiet. It is something I have to get used to.

Music is just wonderful to hear though. I forced the kids to practise the piano. They resisted. My son is so talented. When he started Year Seven, I relented and allowed him to stop the piano. Five months later he started playing. He is so good at playing by ear. He told me the piano is out of tune. I told him to arrange a tuner and I will pay for it if he really wants that. The piano tuner is coming on Monday. Proud mumma. Resilient boy!

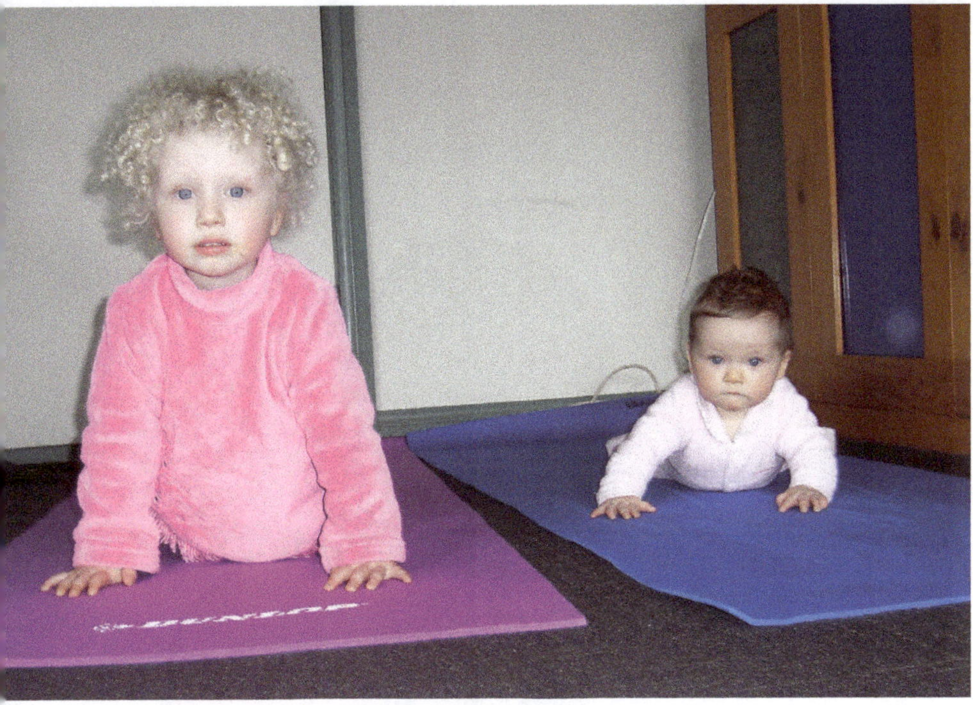

Yoga babies 2013

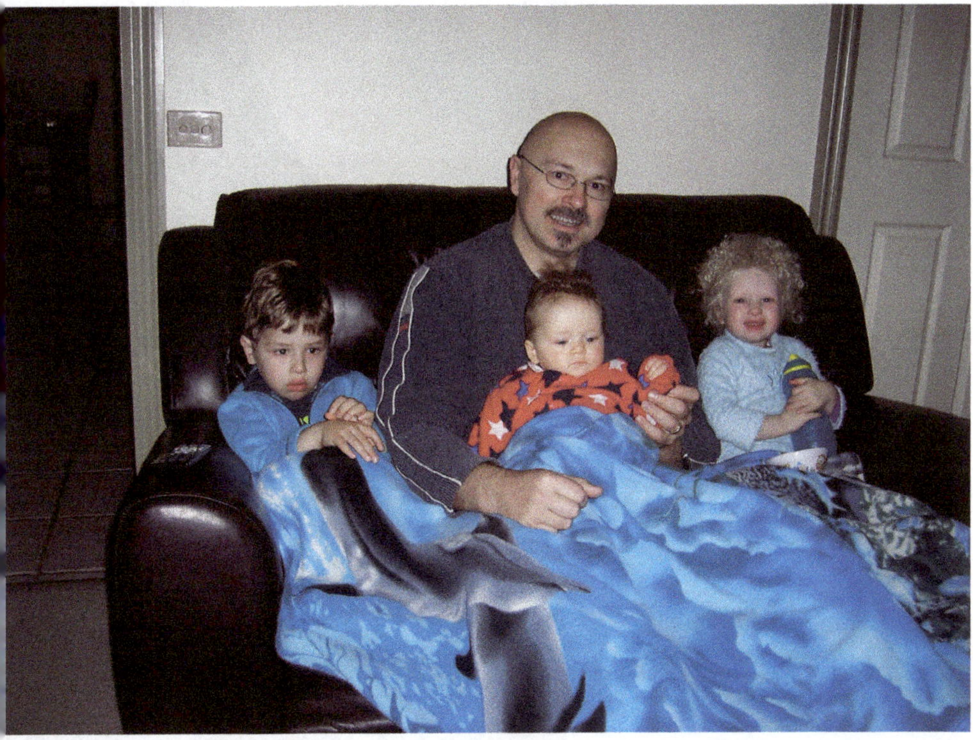

If we ever lost this blue blanket our middle child would be devastated.
10 years later and she still sleeps with this EVERY night folded just the right way.

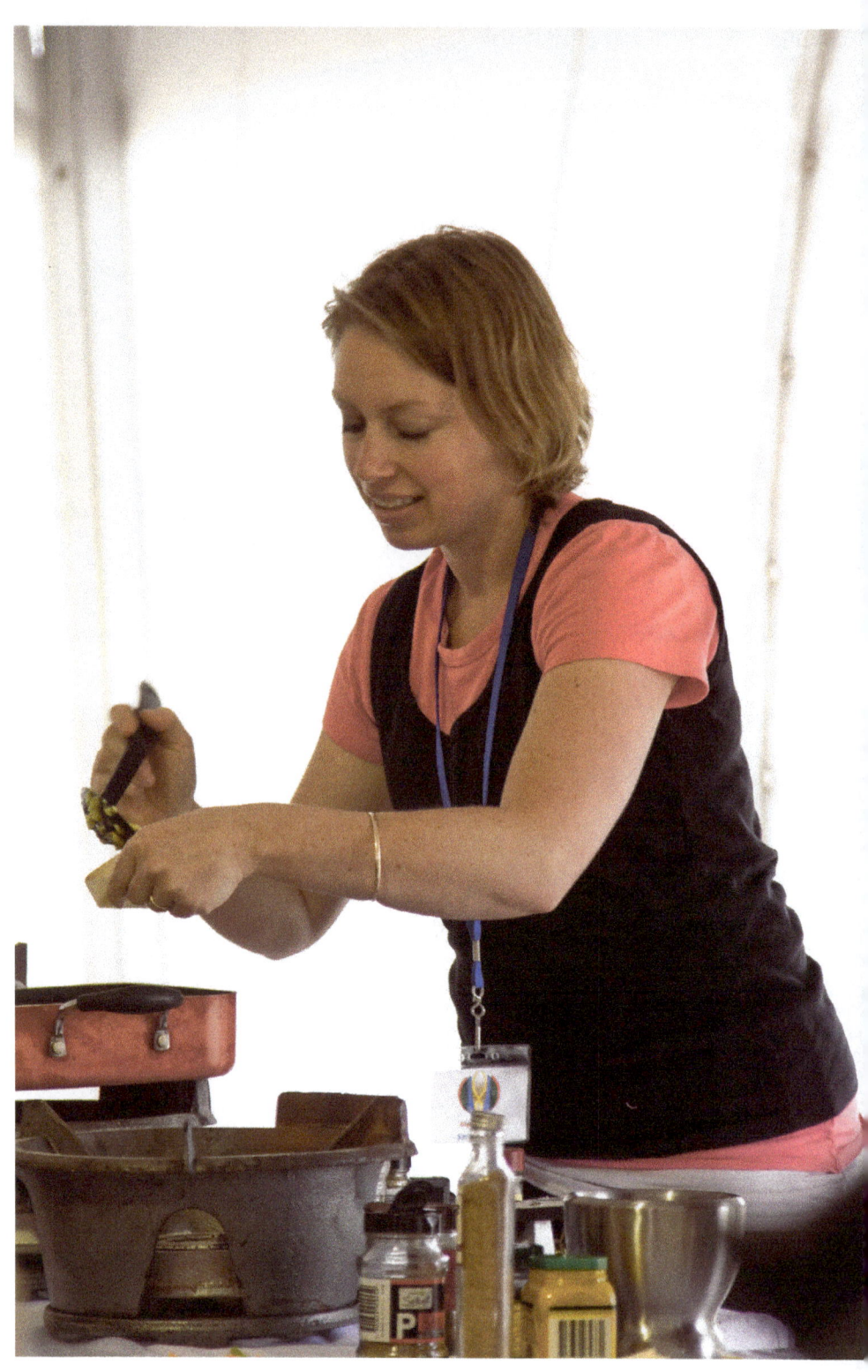
*Me in my element. Teaching Ayurvedic cooking for Yoga Practice.
I shine when I have a role to play.*

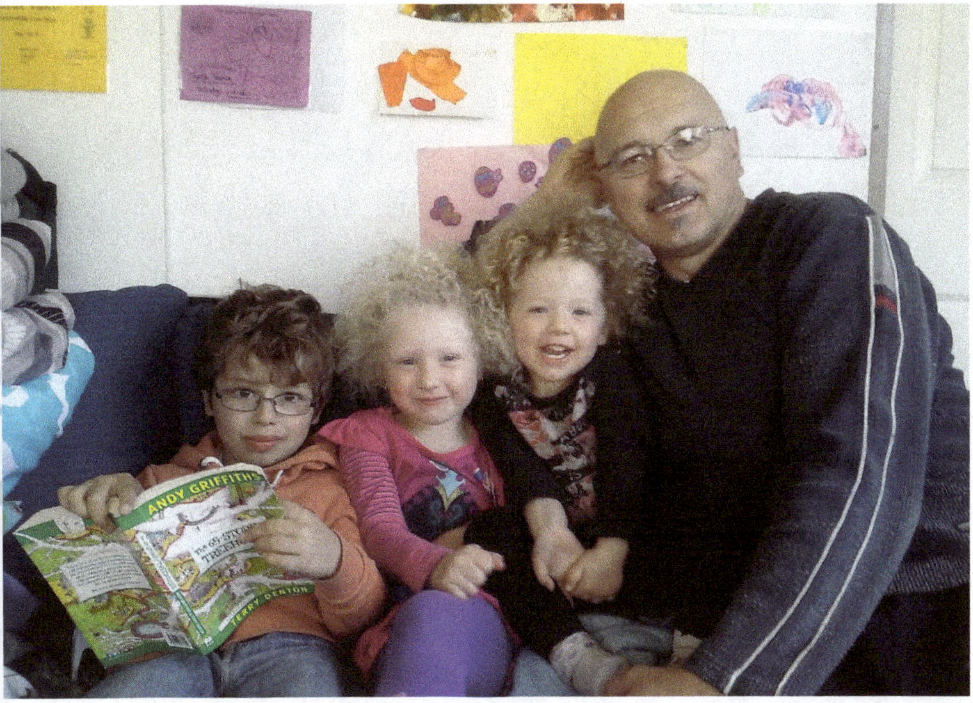

Living in a caravan while we built our home. My son the avid reader. This has never changed.

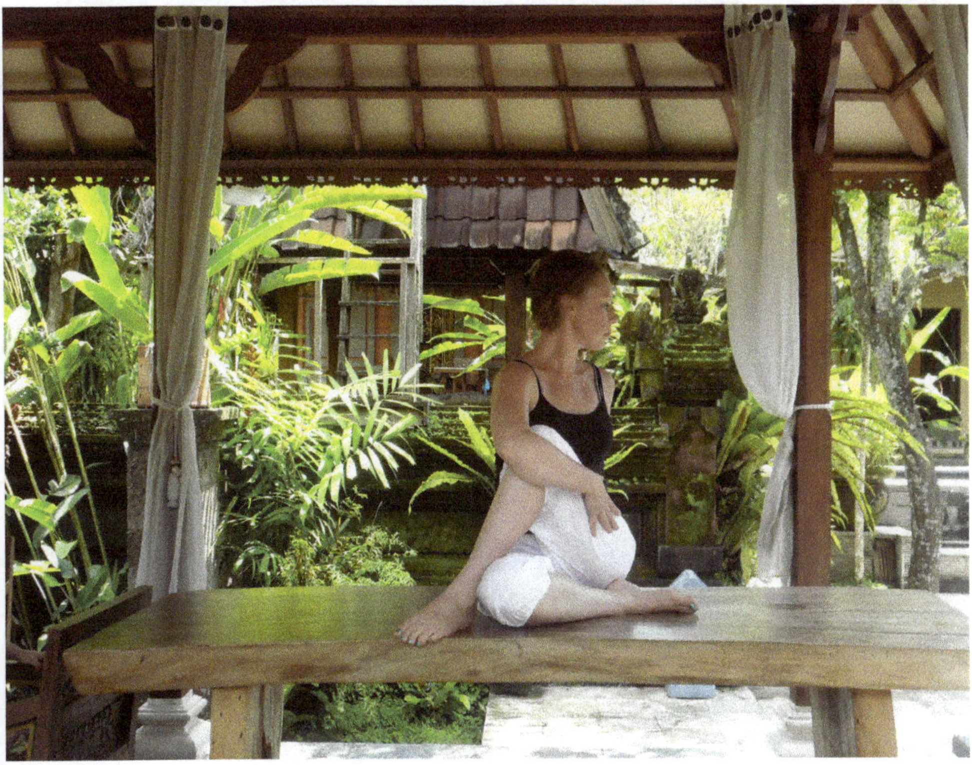

Yoga is my saving grace. And green is my colour.

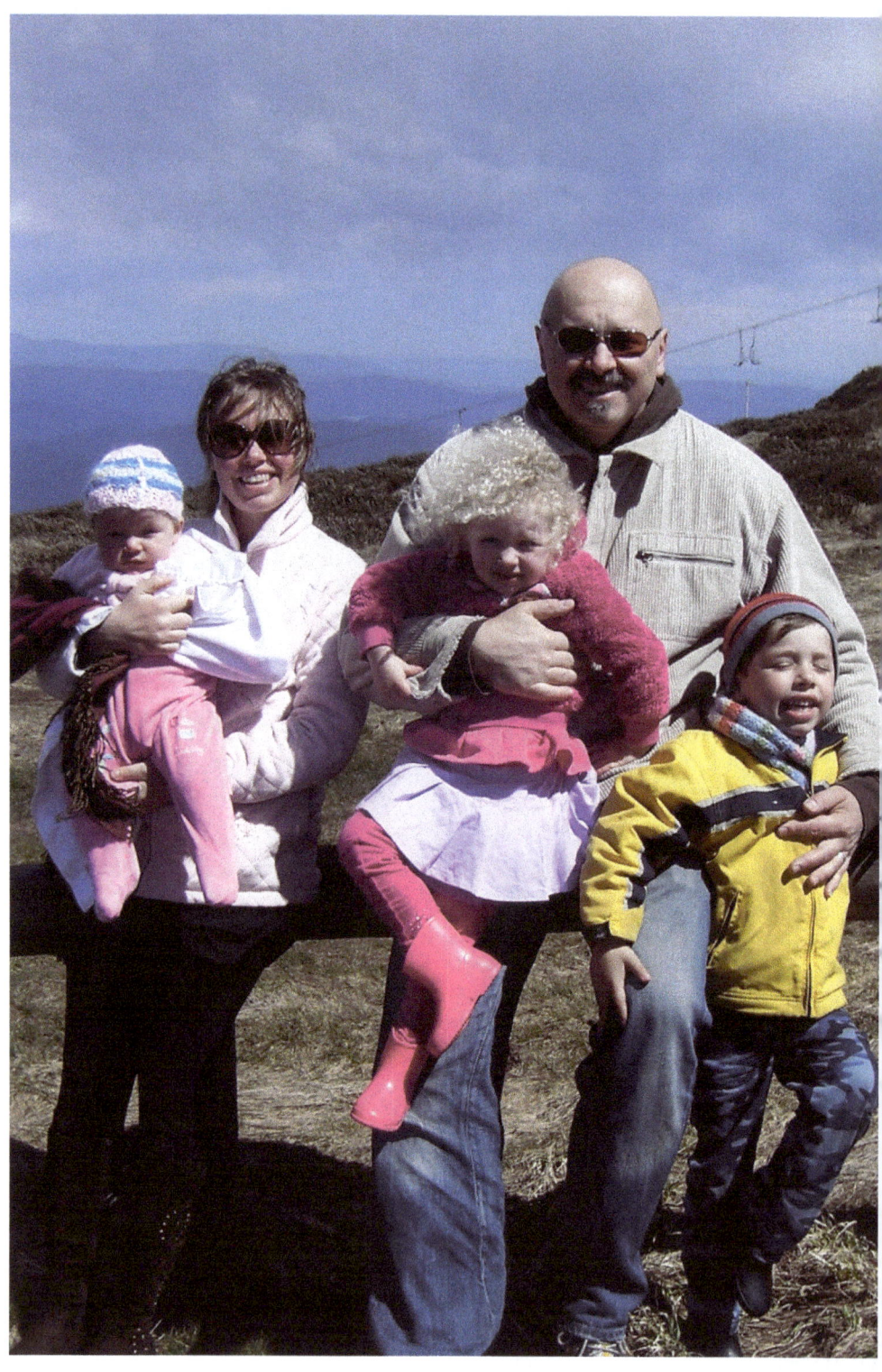

Family holiday to the Snow.
I hate the cold. Holidays were a balance of mother overload and change to routines.
Autism taught us how to holiday quietly.

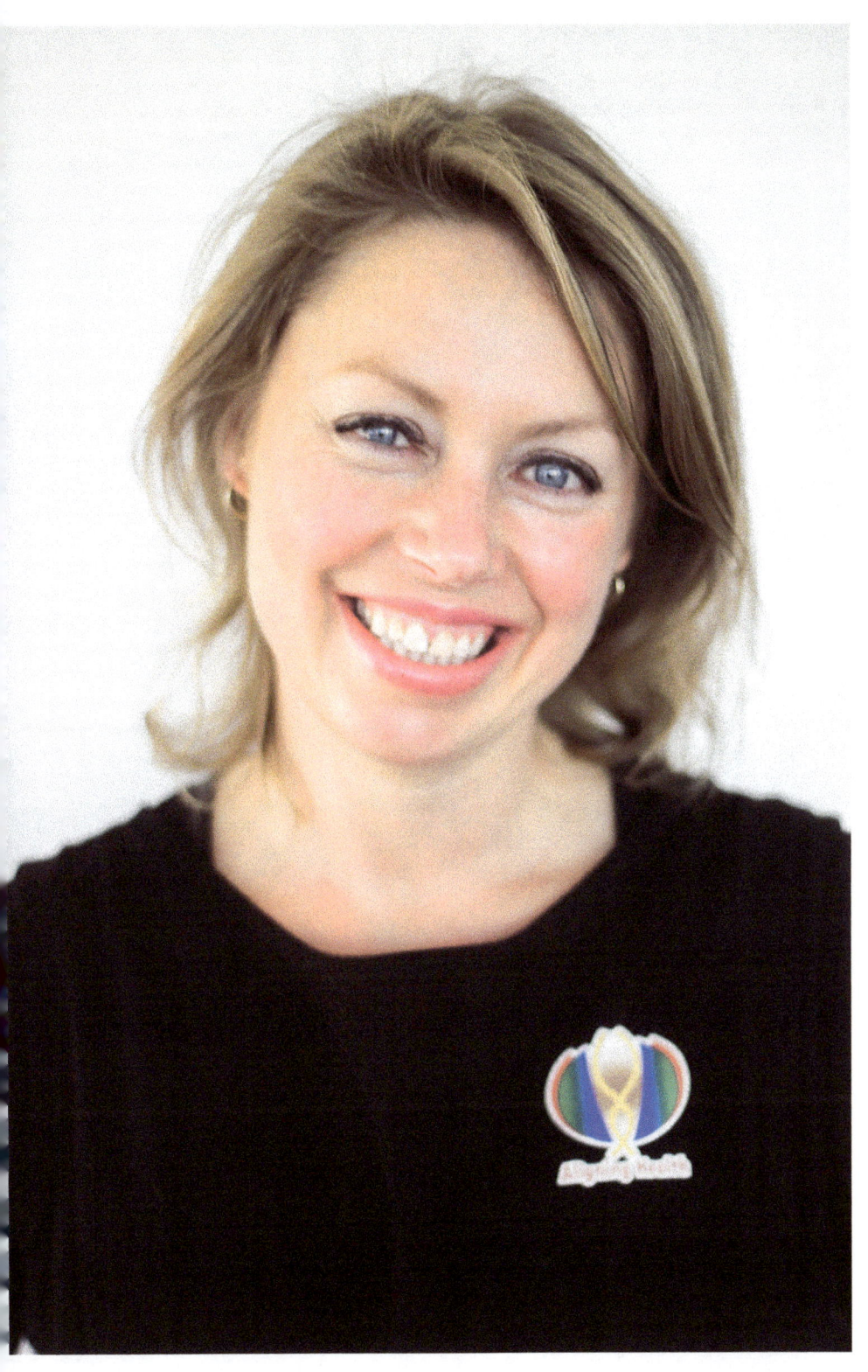
Give me a role and I shine.

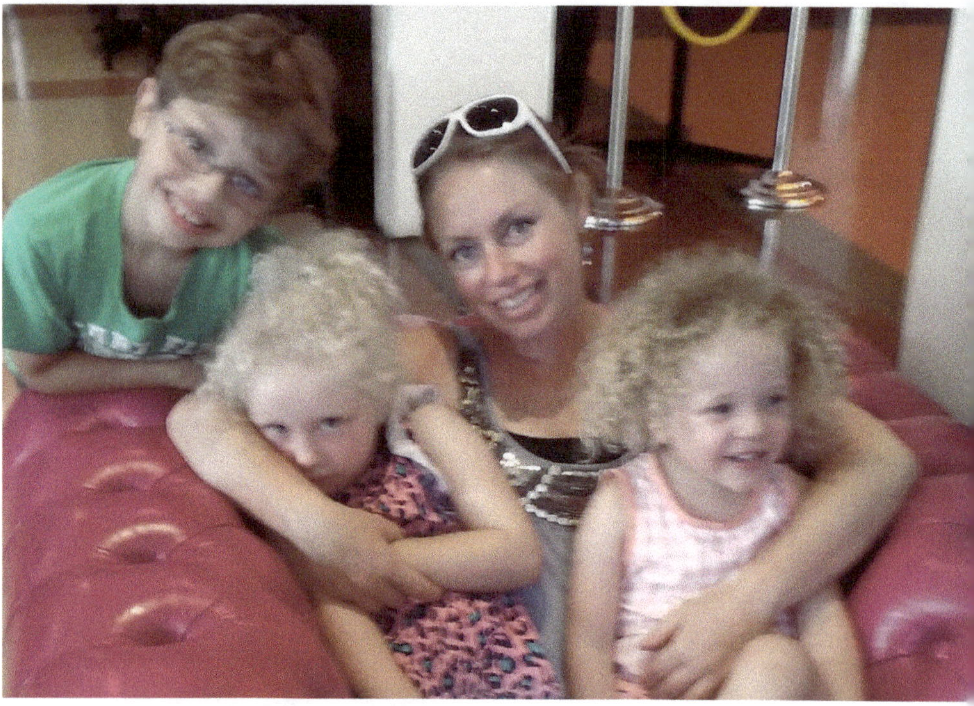

Got em. Every day when the kids were little we would go to a cafe and I would have a coffee at 3pm. This gave me the energy to go into the night.

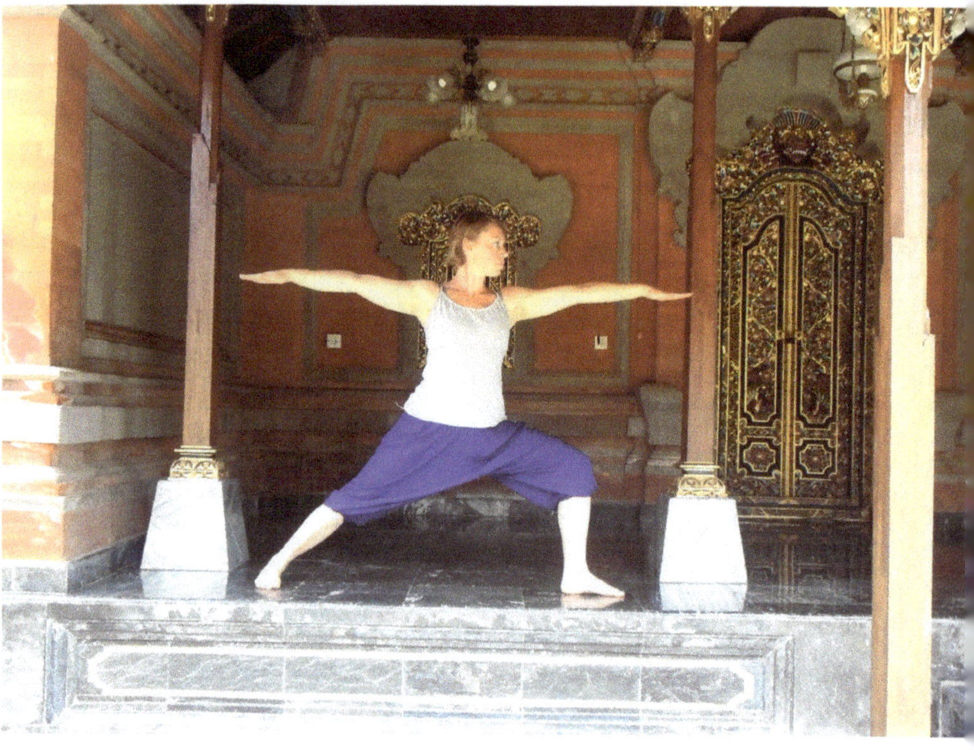

One of my favourite yoga poses. Full of strength

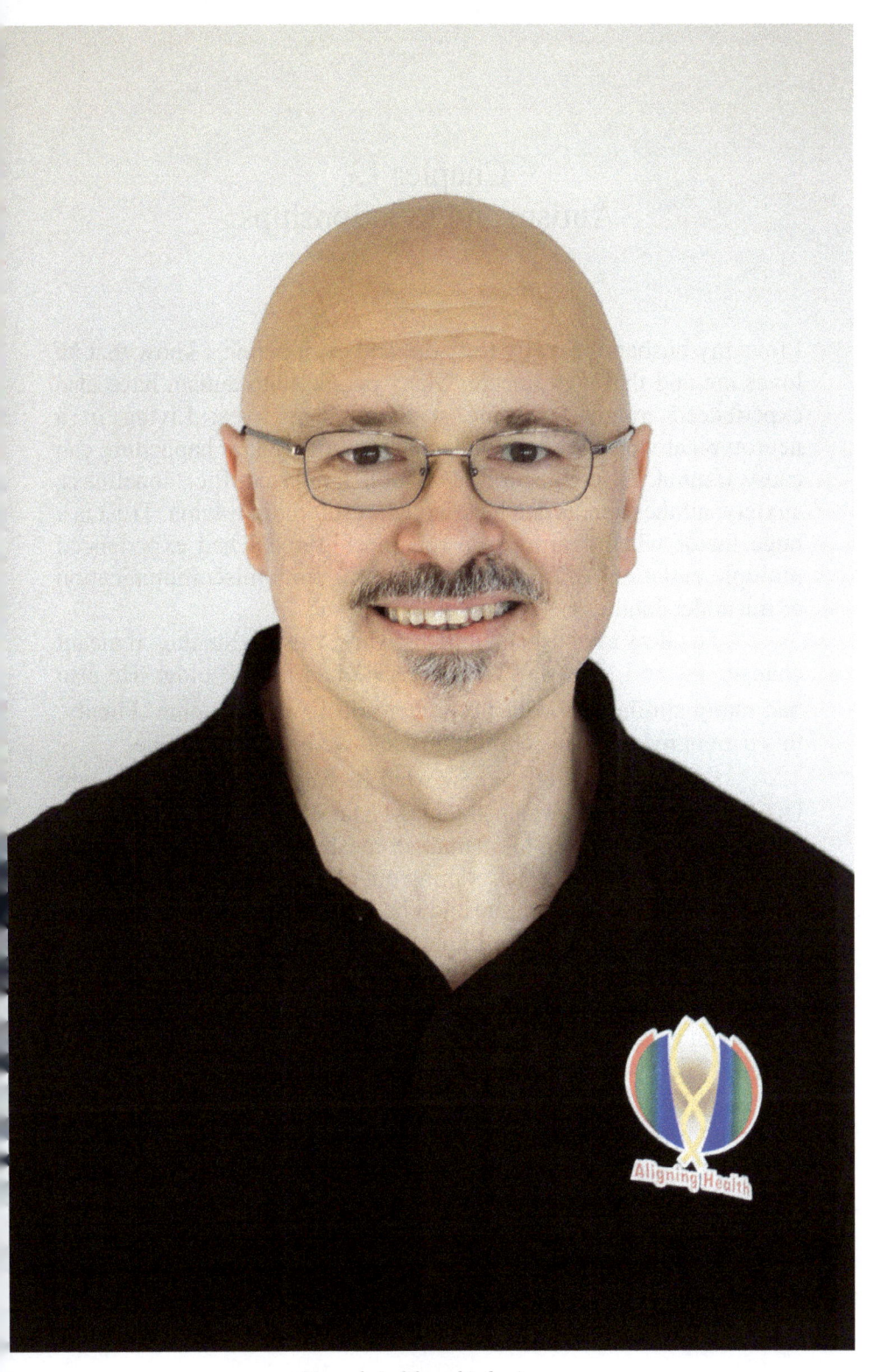

*My rock. In life and in business.
His support and acceptance is never-ending.*

Chapter 13
Autism and Relationships

I love my husband. I really truly do, and even better, I know that he loves me and that it is sincere. Many people with autism have also experienced trauma at some stage of their lives. Living in a neurotypical world without understanding of what is happening can cause trauma. Disconnection at school, family conflict, loneliness, anxiety, all these areas can be affected, resulting in trauma. Trust is a huge factor when sharing in a relationship and I had experienced multiple violations of trust, often stemming from miscommunication or misunderstandings.

To allow my husband into my world was frightening. It meant change. Twice I ran away from him. He is a fair bit older. He also had many similarities with my father and I wasn't coping. Finally, this patient man saw his opportunity and we became a couple.

I'm not too sure he knew what he was walking into though. His family were fairly mainstream. My family was traumatised and had experienced years of mental domestic abuse. When we got together, I was a mess. I was coming out of a fairly substantial eating disorder. I was self-meditating and I had high levels of social anxiety. When I let him into my life, I knew that I could not continue on my path of destruction given how caring and naive I felt him to be.

He held my hand whilst I stopped self-medicating. He helped me to plan what to wear each day. He listened to all my thoughts and worries. There were some things he could not handle. I would fly off tap. Snap. I was gone. I slammed doors. He told me I was not to slam doors anymore. I stopped. We would get ready to visit friends. I would have a panic attack in the car on the way. There were many times I would become overloaded and he would turn the car around and drive back home. This got me into an even bigger state because I was trying so hard to hold it together and psychoanalyse everything beforehand and suddenly, we weren't going. What were people going to think? My self-perception was that I was a bad person. He was exhausted.

When things are good, they are really good. We used to lie in bed on a Saturday and Sunday morning. Most mornings I was too hungover from the night before to get up any earlier and I would be in almost a panic state trying to plan out a weekend that was fun and social. I had this expectation that we had to live life to the fullest, but going on outings was difficult. Most times there was food involved and I was still struggling with the whole food concept. Time and time again my husband would point out that many people had special dietary requirements. My frustration was in my mind. They chose to be like that. I was not allowed to eat certain foods and I was positive people could see through that. I found it really hard to be fake and not reveal my whole life story to whoever we were with. I just felt fake.

So drinking was a great cover. A couple of drinks and I could relax. Drinking and relationships though don't match too well. The get up time on the weekend had to be by 10am. Then hit the gym for 60 minutes. No more, no less. Then come home and try and work out what to do. Too exhausting. Needless to say, most weekends were tense.

Living with someone with a mental illness can be tough. My husband had the ability to be able to see me behind the mental illness. I would often ask him what he actually saw in me, especially as I was emaciated and wouldn't eat when we met. He said he saw someone who really tried and had a good heart.

Living with someone who is misdiagnosed seems unfair. My husband and I have been together for over 20 years. Together we have struggled through anorexia, addiction, depression and then a re-emergence of poor mental health leading to a diagnosis of borderline personality disorder, only to find out the underlying issue is a developmental disability known as autism. We had no idea and we had no strategies to be able to handle this.

One of the things we tried was phone counselling. What a joke. I need to read a situation and a telephone support line is impossible to read. It only made me feel more angry. We tried counselling and I spent a near fortune on private counsellors. Nothing helped and good counsellors are few and far between.

We tried talking. I did and still do continue to debrief with my husband. We recognised the work I was doing in welfare was destroying my soul. My attempt to save the young people from a similar fate to mine was being taken home and drowned in a bottle only to re-emerge again and again and again during discussions. My husband told me he was exhausted.

We agreed I was not the type of person who could easily separate work and personal life so I enrolled in a Graduate Diploma of Education with the intention of becoming a teacher. I completed the course but our lives took a turn and I ended up having a baby, stopping this career progression.

One other thing we agreed on is our misdirected communication. When we are on the same path communication flows easily. More often than not, though, we would be slightly misaligned in our communication. It almost felt like the scales were aligned but slightly ajar. I am very quick to process information and his speech pattern was a little slower. He would take a little longer to plan and I had already made decisions. This led to frustration because he just wanted to finish what he was saying and I found it draining to be on the same path. All my energy was being sapped in the effort to move forward.

A classic example was our discussion over the washing machine. It stopped draining. For me this was a huge issue. I had lots of bookings and was responsible for clean linen as well as navigating the world of school pick up and mother duties. I had pre-diagnosed the issue. Hmm. Too big for me to fix myself. I considered visiting the laundromat. The washing was heavy and half washed before the machine gave way. There was no way I was going to heave all of this into my car, dripping wet.

That morning my sleep had been disturbed. The bird was squawking. The guinea pigs were loud. My baby hadn't stopped talking; thank goodness she was in a happy mood. I told the children I was in the yellow zone and everything was ok, I was just feeling tired. Then my baby snaps. The socks don't feel right. My girl is triggered by my baby. I scoot my baby out of the house on the short drive to take my son to the bus stop. The mood is tense and I can feel everything absorbing into my body. I concentrate on my breathing in an attempt to self-regulate. It passes.

On the way to school my husband rings and my baby talking on the phone is too loud. I am feeling on overload. She hangs up. My baby asks me three times about waterproof shoes, trying to structure waterproofing into her head. It's too much for me. I drop the kids off at school.

I ring my husband and ask him to organise a repair man. He advises me to go to a laundromat in the meantime. This is where I snap. I hang up. I have spent the morning considering all my options. I have spent the morning trying to keep it together and prevent a meltdown from not only myself but the three children. When I try and dismiss the laundromat idea my husband persists in the discussion. I don't have the ability to listen anymore.

The challenge is the dependency I have on my husband. We have a good relationship but he is one of the only people in the world I trust. This makes our relationship all consuming. For me it is fine. I am an intense person, and a lot of the traits of autism revolve around an all or nothing concept. If I walk into a relationship, I give my all. This also means that when my husband becomes overloaded and needs to regather his composure, I can sense it, and there is a negative response from me. Having been told for years that I was the problem by family members also confirms what Sedgewick et al. (2020) suggest in their study of females and relationships, namely that any negative response perceived within a relationship by a female with autism leads to the attribution of blame and poor self-worth, even if it is unrealistic or unintentional.

People with autism, especially females, often blur the boundaries of self-disclosure. In conversations, ideas may be pre-scripted, or the desperate desire to connect with an individual may make the individual vulnerable to different expectations; as suggested by Sedgwick et al. (2020), females with autism put up with unacceptable behaviours or are even taken advantage of due to their desire for acceptance.

Women with autism may also experience deep connections, and possibly a relationship that becomes extremely intense with a co-dependency that naturally develops. In my relationship with my husband, he takes over the parts of life that I find overwhelming simply due to multitasking or consequences of sensory overload. A partner may also act as a gateway to social connection, paving the way for connections outside of the family home, as described by Sedgewick et al. (2020). When I am feeling 'buzzed 'or sitting in the yellow zone I don't have the resources available for socialising. In these situations, my husband is now forewarned that he may have to take over. This negates cancelling and also helps me to navigate my reactions, knowing I can rely on him for an out when I need it.

My relationship with my husband has evolved over time. It has not been an easy journey. We have cried together, talked constantly and re-evaluated what we are dealing with so many times. One thing I have been assured of, though, is his stickability. At the end of the day, he sees me. For that I am grateful.

The communication differences in autism are bound to bring little hurdles into a romantic relationship. What then happens in a family relationship with parents and siblings? Time and time again I read on social media about the inner turmoil of self-disclosure when it comes to family members. Obtaining a diagnosis of autism isn't something that just happens. To even consider moving through the diagnostic process as an adult there must have been some trigger. All too often I read about self-doubt and concerns with how a diagnosis will affect family relationships. Many comments recommend avoiding family. Why?

Family can be difficult. When my children were diagnosed, we were asked to have a parent interview as part of the assessment process. This was then compared to what the therapist identified. What happens when the patient is an adult? School reports, parental observations and reflections help to form part of the puzzle of what is happening for the client. When I undertook a re-diagnostic evaluation, my husband was asked to complete questionnaires. Even though we get on very well his observations and responses were different to mine, remarkably so. Perhaps the client is so skilled in masking and camouflaging even the family don't identify there may be another issue underlying the presentation.

I have suffered very severely with anorexia. I have worked really hard to eat again, but I still have a few hang ups that are difficult to let go of. This led to complications around Easter and Christmas. Big food times for any family. I wouldn't eat chocolate but I didn't want to miss out. I wouldn't eat meat but I didn't want to miss out. Unfortunately, there were limited concessions made for me because my behaviour was considered 'off' and eccentric by my family. My brothers were all big drinkers and huge meat eaters so Christmas featured lots of booze and a few roast meats. I was directed towards the salads, which were often mixed with dressings that triggered my anxiety. To have the ability to communicate effectively against this backdrop of disappointment, disapproval and anxiety was super challenging and after every family event I would have to debrief with my husband. How did I do? Was I ok? Did I say the right thing? Was it obvious I was uncomfortable?

So much effort goes in the preparation of family events and most family events would end up in tears or frustration on my behalf. I just couldn't seem to get in their circle, even though they were my family. My relationship with my mother was always uncomfortable. She had experienced her own trauma and I could see a lot of history repeating for her with my brothers. I tried to be a good daughter, but I could read her too well and my responses were often automated against a backdrop of childhood rejection which made any progress very difficult.

One year I asked her if she would like to come for coffee with me and my children for Mother's Day. She told me she was keeping her options open and said no. I understood her desire to connect with my brothers and her hope they would come and visit her for Mother's Day; but I was there. I was reaching out, and maybe my communication skills did not adequately say Mum please spend time with us on Mother's Day because I would like to see you and I am comfortable sitting in a café with you but nothing else I would find challenging so can we please meet? To be fair, even though my husband and I have been together for over 20 years we still misalign our communication at times, so having a family member with autism requires a little more patience and paraphrasing to really understand the meaning behind communications.

Accepting a diagnosis of autism for an adult within the family can question the whole development of the family unit. This requires a cognitive re-adjustment for the family members and sometimes it is just too difficult for family to adjust their perceptions. They are used to the slightly misaligned conversations, aggressive or passive behaviours, addictive responses and fixated interests of the person in question. To re-evaluate this is a challenge and may threaten the very foundation that the family dynamics are built upon. Hence a lonely path continues with concinnated invalidation.

Friendships outside the family may also present a challenge. Historically it was thought that people with autism did not want to engage in relationships, and the stereotype of the little boy, facing the wall, in the corner, rocking, was seen as typical autism. As we now know, autism is considered to be a spectrum. On that spectrum, people have different needs.

I need social interaction. I find it draining though, as I try and act to a particular formula to appear normal and comfortable. This is a whole lot more challenging without the crutch of alcohol. It means I have nothing to hide behind. It also makes me more abnormal, in my eyes anyway.

Recently we had a group of ladies book the Retreat for a weekend getaway. I opened the fridge. It was full of wine bottles. I take the rubbish away from the rooms, and often I find wine bottles or beer cans people have left from their getaways. This is ok and I am not judging anyone's behaviour. The difference for me is in my inability to self-moderate drinking. I just can't. Drinks have to be even. My whole intention for drinking is based around this concept of relaxation according to the numbers game of consuming an even number of drinks. Autism and alcohol, for me, don't mix. This often makes me stand out. It also means I have to cope on my own. My husband doesn't even get to experience the benefits of me being a designated driver because going out has just become too hard!

Consequently, it becomes difficult to hold on to friendships, and I have experienced this more as I have become older. With my old drinking buddies, things were relaxed and jovial at night; now I no longer have the same lightness. My persona remains heavy. Friendships along the way have dropped off as I struggle to work out what is happening with myself and hide the highs and lows.

A lot of friendships ended badly along the way and this has made it very difficult to begin new friendships without dragging heavy baggage into the new relationships. My bridesmaid was someone who I had considered a close friend. We met during my TAFE years and she seemed to just accept me as I was. This was encouraging and I felt really supported. She also had a best friend and would often debrief about the trials and tribulations of their relationship. That's ok. I was a good listener.

The next year she upgraded her qualification to commence a university degree. I had been told by our main teacher that I would never pass uni so I had no confidence in joining her. I believed this friend was better than me. She found a new group of friends who were also doing university so this meant they were all better than me. We didn't see each other anymore and I was hurt.

A few years later she approached me and told me she missed me. We reconnected. By this time I had partnered with my husband-to-be and she had her own partner. We would spend some weekend evenings together, the four of us. She also had her own group of friends outside our relationship that she would regularly associate with. Her former best friend was long gone by this stage. I could never work out why she never asked me to come along and join them.

Anyway, I asked her to be my bridesmaid. She became the stereotype of the bridesmaid from hell for a bride with undiagnosed autism. She befriended my sister-in-law, who was my other bridesmaid. She was demanding. She was unreliable. One time I summoned up enough courage to confront her and tell her how I was feeling. I was shaking.

On the day of the wedding, she was almost manic, but I felt left out. I was nervous. I couldn't understand her intense moods and was struggling with my own composure. The wedding passed and she got engaged. She asked me to be her bridesmaid and I was so happy! I was accepted! My husband and I threw a thank you party for all the people who were involved in our wedding. She forgot, instead making plans to go out with her other friends. Hmm. She popped over for a minute, ended up having a huge confrontation with my sister-in-law in front of all the guests, and left. I was speechless. I felt it was all my fault.

It got worse. She had developed a friendship with my sister-in-law. She was asking my sister-in-law to do her taxes. Somehow, they got into an argument, and my friend was asking me to get her tax back from my sister-in-law. Somehow, I became the middle person, and this I wasn't going to be: I refused. She knocked on the door of my parents-in-law and fainted. They called an ambulance. They called me. I had nothing to do with anything. Her partner called me. He threatened me. He was a pretty big man and to be frank I was scared.

My poor autistic brain had no idea how things had become so far left of centre. All I know is I had lost a friend, had to explain myself to my parents-in-law to my great embarrassment, and was not as good as my sister-in-law. I just didn't get it. To top it all off, I was left feeling lonely, like there was a huge hole in my heart from our lost friendship.

So, I wrote a letter to my friend. I apologised. In the letter I told her I was sorry and I was always available for her. I drove to her home and put it in her letter box. I am still waiting over 20 years later for a response.

Sedgewick et al. (2020) share a view that relationships for autistic people may be based on activities rather than social sharing. My experiences have been the opposite. I have wondered for many years why the activities I am drawn towards do not develop friendships. Many people with autism overshare and have difficulty with small talk. I agree wholeheartedly with this. Small talk takes time and energy and is just exhausting.

In the past I entered most activities with a hope that they might lead to social connection. The issue is that I see things differently. This can confuse people, as my behaviour becomes easily obsessive and fixated, with a heightened interest in what I am doing. This intensity can be off-putting in a developing relationship. Sedgewick et al. (2020) highlight the behaviours of many girls with autism in developing high intensity friendships with one person. This is evident in both my relationships and my girl's relationships. Full on, intense and with no room in our minds for small talk.

This means our social networks are more limited, and when conflict happens, we tend to take things personally and fixate, not letting go of an overwhelming all-consuming evaluation of what we did wrong. I experienced this in some of my tertiary studies. I started my studies with high hopes and staggering amounts of enthusiasm. When I start something, I complete it. This is the way my brain works and is part of my personality. When I am interested in something I want to share it with the world and talk about it to understand as much as I can to its full capacity! My classmates couldn't cope. I was told by one girl that my energy was too high and I was tiring for her. She likened me to an ever ready battery and told me if I was to be around her, I would have to reduce my energy.

I must have dropped my mask in all of my enthusiasm. I was gutted. I had believed that everyone would want to talk about what we were doing. I had assumed that they, too, would be studying hard and completing assessments; after all, we were paying good money to learn. I was mistaken, and any further conversations with students after this situation were, on my behalf, strained and controlled. Afterwards every communication was evaluated over and over in my mind to assess what I had said, how it was received and if I did ok. My husband once again became my ever-enduring soundboard. The hope of connecting over shared activities was gone.

When we made the decision to move, I made a friend! She was highly academic, as was I. Both of us were very interested in the same topics, wine and psychology. Our husbands also got along well and we formed a good group. To top it all off, we were both very interested and active in social connections and I was thrilled to have met someone who thought along my wavelength.

Sometimes she did things that I wasn't so sure of. One day we were walking along and my mother was with us. She told me she was going to come to my home and fold all my washing. Now, washing and I don't really see eye to eye. I am magnificent at getting it into the machine, but after that it tends to pile up and the thought of putting it away grips me with fear. If you have autism, you may understand what I mean. Anyway, I didn't really want her touching my washing. She might see my husband's underwear and this felt uncomfortable. I said no.

She also wanted to look after my children so I could have a break. My children were my life at that stage; I was loving being a mother and I thought I was coping fairly well. She had these ideas that I would prefer to go grocery shopping on my own without my kids. No way! This was an activity I could endure. It had purpose and direction and it felt like I was on an outing, even if it was just a trip to the grocery store. Again, I said no.

My friend and my mother walked in front of me and started sharing stories about how I wouldn't accept help. I was stubborn. I was a martyr who wanted to do it all myself even if it was the hard way. Not really. Not at all. I was so hurt. Not one of them actually considered asking me if I felt like I needed help and, if so, what that help might entail. Ironically, now that I have my three children diagnosed with autism, I do need help, and I am actively asking for it, but I am finding it hard to get!

My friendship continued. One day I intercepted an email that involved a response to a proposal I had made to our community. It was very harsh and involved a personal criticism of me. I took it hard. I was so upset. I summoned all my strength and phoned her, trying to explain my position. She continued in what I felt to be a harsh response. I couldn't continue in the friendship. A few weeks later she contacted me and wanted to talk. For the first time ever, I refused and ended the friendship. It felt powerful and I was my own advocate. Guess what I did later? I chewed my husband's ear off for weeks on end evaluating every move and re-assessing whether I had made the right decision!

Being unaware that I was part of the autism spectrum tribe was very challenging for understanding relationships and friendships. I took every piece of rejection as confirmation that I was on the deficit model. I really tried hard to make connections but conversations would go dead and I was sure I was the only one that was feeling it. Of course, I would discuss my pain many times over with my husband. He would say that it takes two people to make a friendship and that I wasn't really trying hard. I really didn't understand. I would make an effort, full of energy. For one weekend we would have plans with people on Friday, Saturday and Sunday, then I would be exhausted and it would take me a month to recover. These short bursts of effort were supposed to be precipitated with lifelong friendships resulting in an intimate relationship between families. I always bombed out.

This made me cautious of connecting with anyone; I was coming from a place of fear of rejection. I had waited for my children to be born to connect with mothers 'groups. I had watched my mother and she still saw her group ten years later. It didn't happen for me - I walked in with so much deficit baggage that I was too fearful to connect. The next step was playgroup. In the end I found it easier to chat to the kids. I was mindful of watching and caring for my children and my energy was spent there. Any additional conversation with mothers was difficult to get off the ground. If there was a deep and meaningful exchange, I would go home congratulating myself and fall into a state of exhaustion. Still, I pushed every week, swallowed the discomfort and tried. I had no idea what my husband was implying.

When I began seeing my therapist, I would share with her how skilled I was in masking. No one knew anything unless I decided to divulge. She didn't agree with me. My husband didn't agree with me. They both said I gave off a vibe. I probably had a huge sign on my forehead: Warning! Communication sucking person approaching. I found it all too difficult.

The kids started school. Again, I tried. I joined mothers' groups. I had no idea that meeting multiple women at once was so challenging. My ideas were slightly different. I didn't fit. I assumed it was because I was a new person to the area and put it down to that. However, a year later I was still sitting in the same vibe when newer people than me were accepted into the fold. How did they do that? Just like my family situation. How did my brother get into my in-law fold and not me? That proved it for me. I had a deficit.

One aspect of friendship that has always had me baffled is the reciprocation of groups of friends. I am very good in a one-on-one capacity. When we first moved to our home town, we invited all the neighbours to come for a drink. For me this was common sense. For other people this was unusual. Apparently, it was the first time many of these neighbours had met each other in over ten years of living in the same street. We developed some friendships. I did not expect to be embraced into friendship groups straight away, but it did always baffle me when these neighbours would talk about their friendship groups and never extend an invitation.

I also experienced the same bafflement when I would talk to another friend I met along the journey of life. She would talk about how her friends were all her family and I considered that we were fairly good friends, even close. There were a few times when she had talked about having her friends over and I was also going to be in the area. This was perceived, by me, as an issue for her and the vibe was come if you want to, but we are going to be together and we know each other well.

I also picked up that vibe during other interactions. I had lots of discussions about what was happening on the weekends with friends, but never an invitation to be part of anything. The bafflement comes from my place of open invitation. I would accept anyone at any time. It has been suggested that people with autism share too much. I would share the shirt off my back and I am often confused when others keep their friendship groups, and me, separate.

There is no doubt social relationships can be exhausting for people with autism. Sedgewick et al. (2020) highlight the impact this exhaustion can have on the mental health as a consequence of social mismatch. If we don't fit the mould, we are at fault at an individual level. I knew I would walk into a church and find a group. I could sit up there and recite with the best of them all the prayers and knew by rote the script of the Catholic Church. I could play the game. Except I didn't believe the same way in a God who punishes against the backdrop of an ever-loving God. I had also experienced my own mental abuse from our family priest, which confused me. This was supposed to be a man who represented the God who loved me. I really did believe in the inherent goodness of people and see God in everyone and everything. The tradition of the Catholic Church challenged me and I couldn't do it.

I could also join a netball club. This was the perfect opportunity to meet women around my age. I was into sport and fitness - albeit a bit obsessive in the structure, but I was working on that. I had an injury though. Years ago, I had badly damaged my knees and they had never recovered. If I was to join a netball club there were plenty of opportunities but I would risk serious damage to my knees; and what about the drinking that happens amongst women? This wasn't an option either. So, I was stuck.

What did work for me was distance. Talking over the internet was less intense. Yes, I had to work harder to read a situation but when it became too much, I had the ability to switch off. It also meant I could remain in the comfort of my own home. This was my space and I was comfortable here. I found the social anxiety was not so high and it was easier to relate. Over Covid and during my studies I met a terrific woman who also had some of her own difficulties. We were able to relate on this level and could share intense conversations about our passion - psychology and autism.

My therapist would also challenge my perception of what friendship meant. She suggested friendships may look different for different people. The idea of a group of people hanging out together and having each other's back as depicted in *Friends* and *Seinfeld* is misleading for people with autism. Friendships in autism may just look a little different. It may be that a few solid people who are dependable would fit the ideal of friendship. This fits with Sedgewick et al.'s (2020) idea of people with autism having fewer, but more intense friendships.

What people with autism need to be aware of is the 'burn out' of friendships. Autism may be divided into three levels - social, fixation and rigidity. Relationships, like every other aspect of a person's life, may become all-consuming, and this may lead to exhaustion for the recipient. Having to support a relationship that requires support for psychoanalysis in a highly structured friendship can take its toll, on both the friend and the person with autism.

Chapter 14
Autism Burnout

Many times over I have read that the behaviours of autism become more apparent in women reaching the stage of pre-menopause. There is little known research on this to date. This is hardly surprising given the ongoing stereotype of autism being predominantly a male trait. We women are now being diagnosed in droves, often after years of searching and misdiagnosis from professionals.

When I was younger, I experienced domestic violence in my family, the mental type. This is always subjective and very hard to prove. There are no bruises or external marks. Instead, the internal wounds manifest and cause complications with development. As a child I was a victim of psychological abuse that has led to lifelong scars.

Over the years my strategy to deal with the domestic abuse was to have a physical reaction. There was never an identifiable medical problem, which made the situation worse. I was disbelieved and accused of 'faking it'. However, when I started losing weight, and kept on losing weight, it became obvious that something was wrong, still at the blame level of me as the individual, given the thought that I could eat and if I really wanted to, I would. It was thought to be some kind of manipulation against my family.

I would say my first autistic breakdown occurred when I gave up. I was fourteen years old. My mother was busy educating parents from the church about how to raise teenagers. I was a teenager who was at home on my own, suffering. Recently I had been referred to an eating disorder clinic as an outpatient and was working well with the therapist. My father during that time period was removed from the picture and I was a lot more calm. His constant threat of explosion was removed from the family home. What I didn't count on was my mother's attempts at reconciliation with my father.

When I was fourteen years old, I was done. I could not see a way out of the mess and I felt like I was on my own. My spoons were all used up. Remember people with autism can be masters of masking? I was brilliant at this time. I was camouflaging the extent of my anorexia for fear of being found out. I knew so many tricks now, read many tricks in books and picked some up from watching people in group therapy. If my anorexia was taken away then I would be nothing.

The spoon theory describes this situation beautifully. Christine Miserandino suffered from ill health. She had lupus. One day she explained to her friend the extent of her illness over a conversation at dinner. In Miserandino's theory, we have a set number of spoons each day. Once they are used up, they are gone. This describes perfectly how I feel. I also suffer from ill health - this was the mental kind, not the type identified by a band aid or a plaster cast. It makes it very hard to find compassion or understanding; so Miserandino's spoons theory is a useful way of explaining to people what it's like for me.

My childhood was fraught with an ideology of what perfection looked like. My mother even used to say I was perfect, but my father would say the opposite and somehow it was easier to hear him. I also had siblings who I could not relate with and this negated any concept of me having perfection. Plus, I was already so busy in my head trying to maintain an image that all was ok to the outside world. If I didn't, then why on earth would anyone want to be friends with me?

Every morning when I woke up, to get up, I used my spoons. By the time I had managed the daily meals, assessed the number of calories and dealt with the social environment, I was in a spoon deficit. I could see no way out. My mother, who I loved so much, was busy teaching other parents how to raise adolescents. The spoon deficit became greater than I could handle. My first autistic burnout. Nothing left.

Having autism for me meant that I liked routine. I quickly established the hospital routine. I jab in the morning, a jab in the arvo, a jab in the evening. If the blood came back normal, I would go home. I looked like a pin cushion before I was given the ok to leave, with promises to connect with Child and Adolescent Mental Health

Services (CAMHS). The only issue with connecting, though, was the thought of taking away my safety base, my anorexia and exercise. Not on my watch!

I had previously connected really well with a therapist at an adolescent wing of a hospital that worked with people with eating disorders. She taught me cognitive behavioural therapy (CBT) and it worked a treat! I responded extremely well to the intellectual structure and investigating that was part of CBT. It also meant I got to spend some special time with my mother as she was forced to take time off work and drive me to and from appointments each week. I was starting to take huge strides in becoming well.

Now that CAMHS was involved in my care, the therapist at the hospital rang me one day to inform me, out of the blue, that I was discharged from their service given the complexity of my case and her status as an intern in training. I remember the phone call very clearly. What could I say except ok, thanks. Then I broke. No more spoons at all; and the likelihood of me ever trusting a service such as CAMHS was getting slimmer by the minute.

Between the ages of fourteen to eighteen I was on my own. Resilient and persistent person that I am I fought, hard! Around this time too was when I met the older man I had chased down. We had the most weird co-dependant relationship. I was dependant on him to validate me both internally and externally, especially after my mum had chosen my father over me and my father had spent years telling me how unlovable I was. My spoons were filled by the camouflage of substance misuse and ever-loving promises of nothingness. This helped a busy mind filled with anxiety to float into an abyss of space. Mind you, every time I came back to reality, I absolutely hated my situation. I just had no way out that I could see.

I was living on my own. I was paying rent. I was working. I was eating, barely. I was doing everything that made me look like a high functioning, resourceful young person, with a few exceptions. I was extremely underage to be doing all of this on my own. I had absolutely no support from any extended family member. I was in a vulnerable position, with adult young men at my place on most nights; I was watching my place turn into the party house. I was mistakenly thinking that I had friends and was popular. Obviously, my social graces were mistaken and I would assess, as an adult now, that I was being taken advantage of, a situation that is very strongly cautioned about in Lunden et al.'s (2020) study of females with autism and vulnerability to abuse caused in part by difficulty in navigating social situations.

One day my pretend prince in shining armour was completely inebriated again and started arguing with one of his friends who was even more off the planet that night. Apparently, my prince charming had kissed his friend's sister and the friend was livid. Hmm. This was not a situation I could handle. My spoons were out and I landed smack bang in deficit model.

A few days later my mother dropped by my unit. She didn't do that very often. She found me lying on the bed unable to get up. I spent the next two weeks being a pin cushion in hospital again. Savvy now with the situation, I assured the hospital psychiatrist I would engage with CAMHS this time around and was discharged. My mum dropped me back at my unit and drove home to be with her family. I was still a minor and underage. Needless to say, I didn't engage with CAMHS.

My stay in hospital this time around saw the party house become dysfunctional and people stopped dropping by. This damaged my self-esteem, but the prince came over. I was reassured, and we picked up where we had left off, and it would be another four years before I was able to disentangle myself from this mess of inappropriate social navigation. Unfortunately, I had no one adult or significant other to help guide me along a more normalised path, as every adult I knew had left. A few years ago, I asked my aunty why all my family just left me. She told me they all thought I was being a naughty child.

The possibility of a person with autism presenting as a naughty person may be valid. I was naughty because I refused to comply with the rules my mother put forward at home when I considered returning. By this stage I had been on my own for three years and her rules included a curfew. There was no way I was going to agree to this. I was naughty because I refused to stay with my father and my brothers after my brother repeatedly kicked me in the back one day and my father stood by and watched.

Maybe the behaviour of being disagreeable in group sessions as an inpatient may also be considered naughty. Not following rules generally equals non-compliance. What is difficult, though, is when those rules are not clear, of if they threaten the very structured level of supports that have been set up to cope with anxiety. Unfortunately, most of the times I landed in hospital were when I was at the end of my spoons and unable to care for myself any longer. Being in hospital meant surrender but also a little bit of space from the whirlwind of trying so hard to keep going.

I landed my first stay as an inpatient after the first twelve months of completing my chef apprenticeship. I had a rule. No food. Simple. Period. I was completely and utterly obsessed with food but it was not to pass my lips. Everyone else deserved food except for me. I understand there was no logic to this rule, but that is what it was. I would spend all my free time reading cookbooks. I was, and still am, an excellent baker and would spend hours baking. I had a freezer full of food that I was never going to eat; nor for that matter was anyone else. Working as a chef meant I was around food all day. If one piece of food passed my lips then I would be thrown into torment. My anxiety would be at its peak and I would have to be punished by double exercise or restricting the next day.

Being a chef, I wore a chef uniform in all its splendour. I would spend a lot of time arguing with my head chef about my ability to taste food versus being able to smell food to decipher the taste. I still can't taste until I sit down to a full meal. One day I realised I was in trouble. My chef pants were falling off. These were elastic waist pants of the smallest size, and I could no longer hold them up. Something had to give. I landed in hospital.

It's not that easy though. Ask a person with a set routine to stop and it's impossible. Not only did I have to learn how to eat again, I was being asked to sit. Are you kidding me? I was simply not capable. So, the game begins. I must, absolutely must, go for a walk or do something to be allowed to eat. Hospital staff don't understand this, and just like my family, engaging in such behaviour is regarded as naughty. Not once was I ever asked why. I could easily have explained, such is autism.

Aside from many more hospital stays and a bucketload of counselling for years to come, I did ok. I managed to survive in a neurotypical world, albeit with a bottle or two of wine. Of course, there were multiple friendships along the way that were too intense and ended up in disarray, but I have two qualities that got me through - persistence and resilience.

Up to a point. My next autism breakdown was to take me by surprise and sneak up very, very slowly over a couple of years. I had self-diagnosed myself with depression to understand what was happening. I had everything! An absolutely wonderful husband who I loved very much and who cared for me greatly. I had three magnificent children who I just adored. I had a lovely home. My business was starting to grow. Why was I being so selfish and rejecting all these wonderful gifts? For me it had to be depression.

I was finding it more and more difficult to find interest in anything. I was starting to struggle being a mother and every time I broached the subject with anyone, I was told the kids were just being developmentally normal. All my little mother worries I put down to irrationality and nonsense. I felt like I was fighting to keep my kids connected to my family but I was just treading water that was getting deeper and heavier.

I broke. I was out of spoons. My eating was becoming more restrictive and I could see the re-emergence of an eating disorder. A new term, orthorexia, described me perfectly! This is the inability to eat anything that could be considered unnatural. If it wasn't fresh, I wasn't having it. My food selection was becoming more and more limited and I was very conscious I had three little angels watching me. Too much.

Christmas on our own; too much. I felt the rejection. I felt the abandonment. I could not work out what I had done to offend my family so badly. None of my brothers spoke to me and my mother was too transient. My sister-in-law, once my bridesmaid, had overstepped her boundaries and when I had tried to talk to her I copped it sweet. My parents-in-law told me how she was crying at their family celebrations and how upset she was. What about me? I wanted to scream but the ears were deaf and there was an inability to see the depth of pain that was tearing me apart. It was my fault. I was a failure who had failed my family.

Enter autistic burnout, otherwise diagnosed as borderline personality disorder.

It was getting so much harder to mask as I got older. Little things that were ok before now became sources of frustration, and the tolerance to small talk became even more difficult. Recently I watched an interview on a local television station about the concept of burnout. A doctor was talking about his new book release. The symptoms of burnout were fatigue, losing interest in things that you used to enjoy, skimming instead of reading. My gosh; how relatable was all of this? What do you do when burnout has been going for a very long time?

My parents-in-law visited recently. My husband was unwell. He was unwell for about a month. During this time, it was my birthday. Birthdays are difficult anyway. There is always the fear that family are going to use the opportunity to make contact, which my mother did, and I was in no state to process this. Unfortunately, my husband was still unwell and his idea of getting me a present was food. Then he left for the emergency department. It really felt like the one opportunity for a little bright light was gone. I felt very alone and unwanted.

Not long after that my husband booked in for further investigations. The timing was difficult, and somehow, I needed to manage him, the kids, a business and a hospital appointment on the same day for our girl's broken arm. He had to bring in the troops for help, and he did so in the shape of his parents. They came and stayed overnight, with the expectation they would stay two nights.

When your mind is full, it is very hard to do small talk. My husband was having surgical investigations. I was worried. My baby was clearly having meltdown after meltdown in front of my mother-in-law. The next day I also had two of the children's care plans to advocate for. It was too much. To engage in conversation about how well she cleans the kitchen, or how lovely a cooking pan is, becomes way too much for my mind to engage with.

My girl and I left early for her arm appointment. I just had to go. At the hospital waiting for our appointment, we got on brilliantly! We were prepared, and both of us disengaged from the world for a moment with our headphones and crap on tv. My girl had been really upset before this appointment because her classmates could not write on the plaster. It had a bandage applied to the outside so I advocated well on her behalf and the doctor obligingly wrapped an additional layer of plaster to the outside of her cast. A perfect canvas for signatures. On the way home the vibe changed. She realised she would not be able to participate in the school concert. She was crushed and I copped the brunt of it. She refused to speak to me or acknowledge my presence.

I arrived home. My parents-in-law wanted to know what was wrong with my girl. I wanted to know the results of my husband's hospital investigations. I couldn't talk. I fumed. I held it in, though, and proceeded to make dinner. My parents-in-law prefer not to eat my food, instead preferring to eat their own food. Sometimes this can feel to me like abandonment. We sat for dinner. My son asked for sour cream. He asked again. He asked for a third time, this time in a big twelve-year-old booming voice. I snapped. He broke. When my mother-in-law left for home, she said she was sorry if she had done anything wrong during her stay. I really wanted to cry on her shoulder and say I was overloaded and please help me look after the children, but my parents-in-law don't believe in autism and they cannot see how our children are different. As for me, I am sure I am regarded as a bad tempered mumma.

One of the difficulties with masking is when it breaks. As a mother I need to hold it together, all the time. When I break, I try and tell the kids and explain when I have the ability to do so. I really try and put it into words, but sometimes I don't manage this well.

My girl's broken arm had increased her reliance on us as parents to do the little things for her. Going to the bathroom at night, it was difficult for her to slip the pillow back under her arm for support. Bathing was almost impossible for her to do alone. Both my girls have the most wonderfully curly hair. It is just beautiful, but very hard to manage, and most of the time I am too exhausted at night to be able to keep it in the condition it really deserves. So, I came up with a wonderful school holiday experience! We would book an appointment with the hairdresser for a wash and cut!

The next day we went for our appointment. My baby sat with her head in the basin with a little smile on her face. Her hair was brushed and brushed but due to the fineness and amount of hair she has, it was very dreadlocked. This meant a lot had to be cut. She handled the first hour well. Then, meltdown. To an outsider she just looked like she was in a grumpy mood. As her mumma, I knew better. She was offered a hot chocolate and she shrugged. My chance! I knew the shrug means yes. After one sip of her hot chocolate, she was back. Phew.

My girl was adamant she wanted no part of her hair cut. When the hairdresser suggested layers, she looked at me in fear. So, no layers, but just a little trim. Her first haircut in nearly eleven years! She looked like she was enjoying herself. I kept checking in with our thumbs up, thumbs down signalling system. I didn't read the breakdown.

The girls wanted to buy clips and hair ties afterwards. It was a girls' day, so why not? We went to the store my baby wanted to go to, which my girl had asked to go to a few weeks before. There was something wrong. My girl didn't speak to me. Whilst my baby was selecting hair bows and clips my girl just stood there. She looked vacant. Her gaze was up to the sky. When I am ignored, it makes my blood boil. I held it.

My baby had her counselling appointment. I met my husband at the clinic. I was due to take my girl to her speech therapy appointment. She didn't speak to me the whole time. At the speech therapist I suggested I stay out of the room for my girl to engage without the pressure of me being there. I could hear her. She sounded pleasant and she engaged well. At the end of the session, when I was called in, she went back to her meltdown. I was gutted. We drove home.

By this stage I was hungry. I had just worked six days. I had no dinner planned for me. I was wrung out after four hours of trying to hold my girl's meltdown. My husband was running around trying to do all the household chores and I could see dinner was a long way off. It was getting late and past my pre-determined time for dinner then bed. My son asked me a question about how to cook dinner. I snapped. My son broke. I had been so careful not to talk badly towards my son but my raised voice was enough. Another kid broken.

In these moments it is hard. Sometimes there is an unexpected light. My baby came up to me and looked up into my eyes. 'Thank you for taking me to get my haircut,' she said. My baby. Mummy thanks you for those words.

It took four and a half hours for my girl to be able to share what had happened. I had just started to prepare my own dinner and she came and stood in the kitchen. I asked her if she was ready to speak and she nodded. We moved to the couch and sat. She told me her head hurt from all the brushing. I had missed the cues, even though I had been watching so very carefully.

Later I reflected. One of my secret favourite things to do lately has been to watch the *Housewives* series on Netflix. I am honestly astounded. They get their hair cut and nails painted and Botox and the likes. Personally, I find it stressful getting my hair cut. The small chat is hard. It is a noisy and stimulating environment. I took my noise sensitive child to a place where she became not only hurt because of constant brushing and pulling of her hair, but also had to engage in small talk conversation for over an hour. She melted down. I had already held my own meltdown by engaging with the hairdresser who cut my hair and monitoring my girls. An experience I thought would be fun and positive ended up being so difficult. Debriefing with my neurotypical husband, he tells me I should learn not to get so upset by the kids' emotions. My response: honey, I have autism.

My son is never forgotten. I love him dearly and often become overwhelmed by his demands. His flavours of the month. He becomes so passionate. It is great but with my own busy head I often struggle to combine my own needs with his. The Pokémon names are different sounding. The dinosaur names are unusual and I have to listen hard to process what he is saying. Sometimes I break. One thing that rattles me is the state of the rooms. Never ever doubt a mother's intuition. Sometimes a mother just knows. My son's room was cluttered. There was stuff. He loves stuff. That's ok. If he was a dinosaur he would definitely be a stuffosaurus. He also had old furniture and a mismatched room. I decided he needed a space to call his own. I gave him a budget and told him to research ideas. Then Dad took over and did the room with him. They created a space for him. Ironically the Occupational Therapist he saw also recommended a space just for him, not too overloaded or stimulating.

The space becomes messy, quickly. All of my kids are rotten about putting their things away. Instead, they sit around reading. Sometimes I break. He was due to go on school camp. I told him to pack for camp. I was really worried I would forget, so if he did it now, then it would be done. I came out and he was eating popcorn. Room was a mess. No packing for camp done.

Now, ordinarily, I would be patient and cope with this. Not this time though. I had gone to great pains to book a school holiday experience for him at the museum. What I really wanted to do was curl up for a few days at home, but I had promised and we were going. It had taken me over ten times to look on the system and book the tickets for the family. I kept getting the times confused and was having trouble working it all out. There was the Imax, then the exhibition, then the museum and because of Covid each one had to be time factored in. I was just too overwhelmed. Eventually I managed and the tickets were booked. So, I was already anxious. I had so much to do to prepare the family for the day in town, and myself. My husband tries, but really it is me who organises things. He is good at organising himself and things outside the home. It's just the way he is.

This time I broke. I yelled. I yelled a lot. Can you imagine a veil of overwhelm, that just becomes so big and so huge that it is all consuming and you can no longer think clearly? If things become so greatly disproportionate to the point where you really just want to run away and hide in a hole because you can no longer cope with even the smallest thing, this is it. It's too much. The camp not packed, the room messy, the cleaners coming tomorrow, the museum the next day AGH!

Then I feel like crap. I watch my kids crumble. This is the worst part of burnouts and meltdowns. I fight for my kids and I fight hard. I know where every service for autism is, what their waiting lists are and what their fees are. I advocate so strongly for my kids to access services. I am essentially acting in the role of their support worker because we are on our own and people, even their own father, cannot see what I see. I have studied their behaviour. I have analysed it and formulated plans to support the kids. To the point of exhaustion.

When I was diagnosed with borderline personality disorder it was just me I had to repair. When I was diagnosed with autism on my own, without the children as well, it was just me I had to manage. Now I have four people I have to manage. I also have a husband who I love very much, and who I know loves me too, who is burning out and working with the day-to-day tasks as a reactionary response with no proactivity in sight. Anything he organises for relaxation is away from the family, leaving me with a whole lot of unintended responsibility, and feelings of resentment that activities for fun and enjoyment are not planned with us but are instead away from us. He tells us that if we plan it, or if I plan it, he will gladly come along. Sometimes the planning can be part of the fun. He doesn't see it that way.

I am left in the middle of a mess. A reactive, isolating mess. My baby, who can be so very, very sweet, requires constant guidance and supervision. She thrives on structure and support. This means there is no down time. Our house is littered with emotional zones of regulation, fidget toys, emotion cards and stuff. For me this becomes overwhelming and too stimulating as I make efforts to battle my own autistic stimulations against the needs of each child. The perfect description of an autistic breakdown.

Dragons emerge. Every bloody month. Picture an autistic meltdown. An external display of autistic meltdowns. Now multiply this by fifty. Can you actually picture it? Living with autism is hard enough. Watching every day to make sure you check in and display the appropriate behaviour for the appropriate people at the appropriate times. This is masking at its finest. Imagine once a month having the inability to display appropriate behaviour.

Now picture a room. In this room there are sounds and the sounds are all bearable. There is the sound of the washing machine, the dishwasher, the television is on and there is a radio playing in one of the far-off rooms. Now imagine the screeches of a parrot. Include the squawk of the guinea pig. All this is bearable on a day-to-day basis.

For someone with autism these sounds can be grating. It becomes very difficult to cope. It becomes hard to block out the sounds. Now, throw in some children. School camps, school holidays, and the sounds become even louder. One more thing… throw in post-traumatic stress disorder, and the sounds can put you on guard. You need to be prepared to analyse and understand where the sounds are coming from and when they happen to be able to predict what each one is. That's not all though. For the pièce de resistance, throw in premenstrual dysphoric disorder (PMDD). This final piece of the puzzle makes even the smallest of sounds become magnified a hundredfold. The attempt to cancel out any stimulation becomes exhausting.

I have been gifted with all of these. Autism is often accompanied by comorbidities. With females who have autism, often the comorbidities become the diagnosis and camouflage the autism. This leads to the misdiagnosis many of us older females have received, and results in a bundle of lifetime confusion. PMDD, though, is my ongoing struggle.

My wonderful therapist suggested I have a meeting with a prominent therapist at a women's mental health clinic. This was the first time I had heard of PMDD. Until then I just assumed I was a narky such and such around the time of menstruation. What became apparent during this conversation with the prominent therapist was the absence of these emotions when I was pregnant. They were simply non-existent. Before and after I was like a dragon. I was like clockwork. I would literally feel the aggression come over me like a wave. I hated everything and everyone. Every little thing would throw me and it felt like a dragon was coming out of me, ready to claw its way out. I couldn't control it.

Autism and sensory overload had me melting. I was out of control. The sounds within the room of the bird squawking became like knives tearing at my ears. The sound of my baby's voice was too loud. The heaviness of my son's meltdowns was infuriating. I could look at my children's meltdowns and feel like I was completely disconnected. I was focused on one thing and one thing only. Rip their throats out as the dragon whirled around me. I had absolutely no control of my autism during the periods of PMDD and I would be left shattered and exhausted until I got my period. Every single cycle.

For years I had been so proud of my drug free lifestyle. This included pharmaceutical drugs. When I was very sick with anorexia, I had been prescribed a cocktail of anti-anxiety, antidepressant and anti whatever else medication. During the experience of my autistic breakdown as an adult I was sedated. The silly therapist at the eating disorder department of the local hospital, apparently an expert in eating disorders, saw borderline personality disorder as prominent and promptly had me medicated. I was a walking zombie. So I was really, really proud to get off medications once again.

But the dragon lurched every month and I was getting exhausted. The prominent therapist prescribed the pill to regulate hormones. My gosh. It was awful. One thing that keeps my husband and me going is our healthy private life. My reaction to being on the pill extinguished any need of intimacy and if there was, it felt like a muffler was placed on top. The pill was not for me and unfortunately it didn't help the dragon.

Six months of cycles later and I was wiped out again. On top of learning about my own autism I was busy researching and preparing a case for my children's individual characteristics of autism, ringing service providers, studying, managing my emotions. Stop. Too much. Against my desires I agreed to trial another antidepressant that targets women in menopause. Again, to no avail. Medications and me simply don't mix. I get no results.

There has been limited research to date on autism and menstruation. Given the history of misdiagnosis and the late diagnosis of women who have autism, this is hardly surprising. Many services are geared towards early intervention and the emergence of late female diagnosis, although increasing in numbers, is still in its infantile state. I experience autism on steroids around that time of the month. Any hope I have of masking is gone. My energy is sapped and to top it all off I have this dragon that I wrestle with, which feeds on overstimulation of sensory sounds.

I don't know what to expect with autism and menopause. I am working really hard to keep balanced. I do this by learning what I discovered during Covid lockdowns. I am not superwoman. I need down time. Sometimes the down time is so refreshing it is hard to get going again and I need to keep a check on that and not let that dark dog of depression creep up and overtake me. What I did discover in Covid is that it is ok to take breaks. This was compounded even further by my inability to work to the same intensity due to my children. Recognising the symptoms of autism in my children has meant that I could no longer apply the same passion and commitment I had to my business. The children have, and always will, come first, to the best of my ability.

To keep balanced I apply my knowledge of yoga and Ayurveda. Ayurveda for me has been an absolute godsend. It has, for me, given me rules to live by. It has helped me to understand how I am feeling physically and the impact it has on my food and lifestyle. Using the knowledge of Ayurveda has helped me to understand the qualities of autism and the qualities that exist in me.

Ayurveda is Indian science. It is based on a practice that believes everything in the universe is made up of five elements, these being space, air, fire, water and earth. We are a combination of all of these elements and the ratio of these elements is what makes us unique. These elements have particular qualities or characteristics. The words to describe space and air are things like movement, cold, dry, unexpected, fear, lightness and subtle.

Autism is predominantly composed of air and space. Air and space have no grounding. It moves. This is the job of the air and space. It helps to move things through the spaces of our bodies and minds but for me this movement gets aggravated, quickly.

In the yoga world it is believed the mind moves. The thoughts that move through the mind may cause disturbance. Apparently, I have suffered anxiety all of my life. Who knew? I had thought it was depression. It looked like aggression. It was anxiety. I had a fixed belief. This may also have been one of the reasons I was misdiagnosed with borderline personality disorder. I had strong, very strong ethical beliefs and a strong sense of justice. I would fight for justice and become fixated on the notion of right or wrong. I was completely attached to the way things should be.

Yoga and Ayurveda would suggest the mind has grasped on to an ideology of attachment and the inability to just see things as they are causes conflict. You betcha! The requirement to have life operate in a routine also sits within this realm. I am not attached to things, but I am attached to ways of operating. A sleep in on the weekend sends me into chaos because it moves against that set routine of the day, my fixation of what the day should be.

The fixation of the mind on the concept of set structure is also a delusion. There is absolutely no evidence that sleeping in is going to throw a day into chaos. Existing in this state of mind is a delusion that prevents living in the moment. The air and space that is required to move becomes stagnant. The mind is stuck. This results in suffering as the mind becomes poisoned.

The challenges to change this fixation are real. I get comfort with routine and structure as well as hating it at the same time. If we go on holidays, I am the one who jumps out of bed to go and workout so my mind can be mentally prepared to cope with the demands of the family, or even just the activities of the day. Even when we try and have romantic holidays, I need that structure. As limiting as this delusion and attachment may be, it keeps me settled. The more I work on challenging these ideologies, though, the less stuck I will be. They truly do cause suffering, and peeling back the layers of attachment bit by bit helps to bring life into the present and move against the veil of disillusionment.

Ayurveda teaches the ideology of balance. We need air and space to exist. When there is no space, there is no movement. The very first piece of air and space is life energy. When life energy is gone, we are dead. It really is that simple. This is why it is so critical to eat food that has life energy and is not manufactured. If you are vegan, be vegan by eating real food, not manufactured food. If you eat meat then eat real meat and not precooked frozen meals from the freezer aisle. If you are vegetarian then soak some lentils instead of cracking open a can. Life energy is critical for good digestion of both mind and body.

Sometimes this air and space needs a little more support though. Regardless of the amount of elements of space, air, fire, earth and water we have in our body, we may be born with those ratios a little out of balance. We may even find those elements move out of balance through lifestyle and diet choices. Ayurveda needs to balance space and air.

Chapter 15
Living With Autism - Rewriting The Story

Autism is diagnosed by challenges with social skills, communication, repetitive behaviours and sensory stimulation. My challenges with autism are all of the above. Sounds become too loud. I become so aggravated by sounds. My husband and I still have a major disagreement in our life: I swear there is a generator I can hear at nights; he can't hear it. My hearing is so sensitive it throws off my ability to relax and I feel tension moving through my body, constantly. Both yoga and Ayurveda philosophy believe we make meaning of our world through the sense organs. Ironically, hearing is associated with the element of space. I have absolutely no space in my head when there is an aggravation of sound in my environment.

My baby does not stop speaking all day long. My son speaks about subjects he becomes fixated on. The fireplace has a fan that is noisy. The fridge hums. The dog scratches at the door. One more sound and I will crack. I have to balance my autism using my knowledge of yoga and Ayurveda. Ear plugs. One of the best inventions of all time. I think I have tried every pair of ear plugs under the sun. Some are aggravating. I can hear my breathing when I wear them. Some block all sound and it becomes frustrating when I want to hear my children. I still have yet to find the perfect pair but I can guarantee one thing, they work to take the edge off the overstimulation of sound. For that moment they can be so beneficial to prevent a meltdown that every penny spent, and every pair trialled, is worth the effort.

Some people with autism become overloaded with touch. My son likes textures. We both hate tightness. We choose to wear elastic waist and loose clothing. Both my girls become extremely aggravated by socks - yup, socks. It can take us so long in the morning to leave the house because of the feelings of socks. My baby says 'the socks are misbehaving again'. We have tried to reason with them. My husband, ever the science teacher, tells the girls that five minutes of wearing them will make them forget their aggravation. Most of the time the aggravation is so high, though, that five minutes just doesn't even get there. So we have invested in socks made of bamboo with no seams. We buy clothes that are not scratchy and we try our very best to draw, write or say what aggravates us at that particular time.

When my mind is busy, I feel cluttered. I assume this is a sensation that neurotypicals feel as well. I'm not so sure it makes them want to rip their hair out though, and sends them into an anxiety attack. My mother used to teach us to clean the bench. She would say she could cope with mess as long as the kitchen bench was clear. I am similar, magnified by one hundred. When the rooms are messy, I panic. When the kitchen bench is not clear I panic. Kids' shoes, scattered books. It feels overwhelming and I become panicked. My head is already so busy and I'm concentrating so hard on keeping the sounds in check and my behaviour under control that I cannot seem to handle stuff. Stuff. Our world is littered with it! When we lived in the caravan whilst building our home with a 12-month-old, a two-year-old and a five-year-old there was less stuff and I really did feel less panicked. Now in our home, there is stuff!

Many people with autism are sensitive to smells and tastes. As a young person I worked at Klein's jewellery store in Eastland. The job was simple. Retail is not my forte though. My colleague would have a banana for her morning tea. The smell would be overwhelming in the store and make me feel nauseous to my very stomach. My girl cannot tolerate particular textures in food. Smooth textures make her choke. Before we knew about autism, we would yell at her for not eating. Now my husband and I understand. It is a sensory issue for my girl that she is unable to control at this stage.

Understanding the senses and the effects on the body and mind by knowing yoga and Ayurveda really helps. We become more equipped to intervene and reduce the chances of burnout. We are still learning in our family, but more and more we are recognising the importance of understanding the self and applying life knowledge which is the true meaning of the word Ayurveda.

Running my business means I have the opportunity to work with some amazing people and share their stories. One of the strategies for autism I was hearing about repeatedly was heaviness. Applying my knowledge of Ayurveda and the lightness of space and air, this just makes sense. Autistic nervous systems are continually on high alert and sensory stimulation sometimes feels like bombardment. Heaviness helps to counteract this lightness and for me it brings wonderful relief. After a really busy period working, I kept hearing about these weighted blankets. I was feeling a little wrung out so I took off up to our local shops to buy one. I measured the size and estimated 7 kilograms would be sufficient. Arriving home, I unwrapped it and sat under it. Oh my God. It was bliss. I lay down. Hmm. It could be heavier. My son lay under it and his face showed just pure relaxation and release. That was it for me. I raced back up to the shop, much to my husband's bewilderment, and bought the biggest size available - 9.5 kilograms. This has been placed over the top of my three other doonas on my side of the bed. It is so heavy I can hardly roll over but I love it.

I get super duper cold. Anything hot is pure delight. Really, the hotter the better. I get very addicted to patterns of behaviour, which is one of the reasons why I will never again touch alcohol and I need to keep a very careful check on my level of exercise. I have got one behaviour I indulge in. Coffee. Ahh. Strong coffee. Warming. From the same place. Every day. Only one a day. And hot, extra hot. My standing order is a large cappuccino extra hot.

I love the heat bags. My family call them warm ups. A lukewarm heat bag is a disappointment. I like them steaming! So much so last year one of them caught fire by accident. And a shower. Hot. Steaming hot. Unfortunately, in Ayurvedic practice it is recommended to have showers lukewarm, particularly as my natural constitution has heat. A hot shower feels like it is a hug and melts away all my pain and thoughts.

For my birthday this year the kids bought me an Oodie. I had looked at these great big blanket-like, weird, triangle-shaped, jumper-type things and showed no interest. When they presented the Oodie to me, I put it on, for their sake. Oh my God! It was heavy. It was fleecy. It was warm. It was also coloured like a huge pink donut but I put that visual aside. I looked forward to the time of the day when I could slip off my day clothes, let go of the demands of having to mask and put on my Oodie, heat my warm ups and somehow slide into the weighted bed.

Space and air have the qualities of dryness. Looking at the practice of balance, dryness is balanced by moisture. The moisture also has the added benefit of heat when applied warm and oils that are warmed are more easily absorbed into the body. When I was unwell with anorexia, and truthfully up until eight years ago, my diet was controlled with a complete absence of oil or sugar unless I was drunk or premenstrual. An amazing Ayurveda doctor asked me to put both back into my diet. I did so with complete trust in the doctor as it took every single ounce of my courage to follow her advice.

I also began to massage oils into my body. The oils are warmed. The selection of oil is based on sesame. Sesame has the qualities of sweet taste with a heating effect and is used to help calm the nervous system. My knowledge of Ayurveda has also helped to select specific oils which are made with herbs that help give an even deeper response. Ayurveda oils are made following a time-honoured process. The herbs are prepared into a powder known as a churna. The powders are then cooked into a decoction, similar to the way we may make a chai from spices by cooking it and reducing it to a potent tea. The solution is strained and the decoction is cooked with sesame oil over a low heat for twenty-seven days until the water is removed. This makes a very potent and strong massage oil. When I heat the oils, the herbs are absorbed through the skin. The very act of massage helps to calm the breathing and bring some attention to the part of the body that is being touched. Even better, it is anti-ageing and the wrinkles I am noticing get a little extra attention!

I also use a product called ghee. This is simply unsalted butter cooked until the milk solids have been removed. Ghee in Ayurveda is widely used and is said to be highly beneficial for the digestive system. Ghee is used to nourish all the tissues in the body, which is really useful for a client who has experienced an eating disorder for more than half of their life. It is calming for the mind, which is essential for a client who suffers with anxiety. So in a nutshell, ghee is a great substance for autism and for me. As someone who has had an eating disorder I was deathly scared of ghee. I have noticed though that my digestive system has improved and I have not put on weight. The theory that ghee will flush out of the body when ingested warm remains true for me. It has to be used warm and not cold. Again, this meets the criteria of warm and heavy to help balance the qualities of dryness and lightness associated with an excess of space and air.

Excess of space and air is all about an abundance of movement. Put simply, there is too much. In today's world we are fooled into believing we can multi-task. Yoga would suggest we have the ability to do only one thing at a time; however, because our minds move so fast, we may be misled into believing we are capable of doing more than one thing at once.

For me, with autism, this multitasking is impossible. The abundance of different thoughts, sensations, and 'have tos' becomes overwhelming. Getting three children prepared, considering the needs of a husband and trying to take care of myself ultimately led to a meltdown. Too much, too overwhelming. The concept of multitasking negates the ideology of single pointed consciousness and being in the moment. Yoga practice reduces the fluctuations of thought according to the Sutras of Patanjali and therefore the action of multitasking has a dire response.

Autism strategies for behavioural support advocate the implementation of structure and routine. Autism is essentially a different way of operating in the realm of communication, often becoming fixated with behaviours and sensory overload. Structure and routine help to provide a systematic boundary. The objective of speech is movement. To understand speech and communication there has to be movement of the information into the brain. This is controlled by the elements of space and air. Interpretation of the world around us is conducted through sensory experience. This is essentially controlled by the movement of the elements of space and air. To put it simply, space and air, known as the Dosha of Vata in Ayurvedic terminology, are seen as being too high on the balance of scales for most people who have autism.

To place routine and structure within a lifestyle assists in the grounding of space and air. When I was a child, I would panic when I had choices. My mother used to allow us to get our own lunches on the weekend. The choices were usually two-minute noodles, hot dogs or meat pies. How on earth was I going to make the correct choice? I wanted all of them! The choice of spreads on my toast would throw me into a cognitive spin. Do I choose vegemite or peanut butter? One day I changed my mind mid spread and ended up with half vegemite scraped off and then topped with peanut butter. I don't recommend this combination! Not only did I have to choose what to eat, it had to be even. If I had two slices of toast and I wanted another one then I would have to have four, even if I wasn't hungry. This, in my state of anxiety, kept things safe and clean. This reasoning is also one of the reasons why I am careful never again to touch alcohol. If I have one drink it has to be two. It cannot be three or five because my logic considers it dirty and unfinished, no matter how illogical it may seem to others.

Routine and structure also exist within the day-to-day operations. As a child I found the school holidays hard. They meant a change of routine. I had to plan and think about what I was going to do on the school holidays and even the weekends to make sure I used the time effectively.

I see this in myself to this day. Recently my children went back to school. For the last five weeks I'd had one of my family members at home with me. A husband with stress resulting in pain, a daughter with a broken arm, a cough from the other child during Covid time. There was no down time. On the last day of the holidays, I wanted to do something special but it had to be the right thing and it had to be something I could tolerate because, quite frankly, I was exhausted from being around people and looking after their needs for so long. This sent me into a panic. I could not think of the perfect thing.

Every weekend we go through this scenario. Sometimes people say to me: take a break. Enjoy a day off. What they are not comprehending is that the choice and lack of structure that comes with having a day off makes me feel lost. Most of the day is traumatic, with constant planning running through my head in the days leading up to it, constant evaluation during the day, and regret that I didn't do what I wanted to do the day after. This sounds illogical but it is so real! One of the benefits I find of study is the structure, even if the study itself causes stress, because it is something I enjoy, am interested in, and it means I don't have to plan the weekends.

All of these examples are attributed to my autism, and the mental health issues that accompany autism, namely anxiety and post-traumatic stress disorder. In Ayurvedic terminology these examples are diagnosed as a state of Vata imbalance caused by an excess of space and air in the system and a mind that is constantly active and analytical leading to a state of rajas - a stimulating state of mind.

One of the first steps to change is awareness. I am going to counteract this statement. One of the first steps to peace is through awareness. Let's be really clear. Autism is not a deficit. It is a way of existing in the world that is not adhering to the neurotypical definition of relating. There is nothing wrong with a person with autism. However, when there is not a diagnosis of autism, but a display of behaviours that are assessed through the neurotypical lens, then issues occur.

My baby is so loved. I have always struggled to understand her behaviour. I have been vocal about this and asked for help from people and professionals for years. Her behaviour was deemed to be developmental or part of her personality. I continued to flounder and her behaviours became more extreme.

When there is no routine and structure my baby is so hard. Recently, during the Covid lockdown in Victoria, my husband and I threw our hands up in despair. We cracked. There was nothing we could do to help her settle. Her behaviours were setting me off. The other two kids were being set off. My husband was lost.

We played board games with her that she wanted to play. Meltdown. She stomped off yelling. We cooked with her. We didn't cook the way she expected. Meltdown. We asked the other kids to get some exercise and jump on the trampoline with her. Meltdown. They didn't play the way she wanted them too. This was happening over ten times a day. Every day. We made a decision. Victoria was in lockdown. I was beside myself. My baby was in misery. We grabbed the dog and all five of us jumped in the car and drove half an hour to a secluded playground. Ahh. Freedom! She was great. The kids all played and we had a ball.

My son created some huge dinosaur footprints in the bark, a sign of his latest obsession. They looked great. We all walked over to admire them. My baby kicked them and covered them up.

My son was distraught. My husband and I just looked at each other. In a split second all that relaxation that we had experienced vanished! We put the baby in time out. I sat with her whilst my husband tried to console our son. My baby retreated further into her meltdown. I was starting to meltdown but I had to hold the space for the children. We now had two very different presentations of autistic meltdowns. One child was retreating and pulling away, saying things like 'this always happens' and internalising the events. The other was kicking and refusing to sit, screaming, with a scowl. Both the kids are diagnosed with autism level 2. Both of the kids display very different behaviours of autism. And myself, my autism comes out in aggressive, anxious behaviour, where anything in my path becomes attacked verbally.

My husband and I had a choice. Persist with trying to reason with our baby and wait until she comes out of her meltdown and may even apologise to our son, or drive home. We drove home. As soon as we got home, I rang the principal of my baby's school and asked if she could go to school for the remainder of the lockdown. She agreed, no questions asked.

Next step, I told my husband, and his relief was evident. Finally, I took a breath and told my baby. I was really worried she would interpret this action as a deficit against her character. I was very aware of her becoming more aggressive, or even problematising her. I had experienced enough rejection because of my own autism from my family of origin and I was trying to be so careful that she wouldn't interpret this action as rejection. She simply smiled.

Happily, she started to get her uniform ready for the next day. She prepared her own lunch. She found her shoes. She went to the whiteboard and wrote her schedule for the next day. She was as relieved as we were. My baby could now see structure. This is what she knew. Now she knew how to play the game. This is a clear example of excess of space and air and an imbalance of Vata. It demonstrates how important routine and structure may be to help a person with autism.

All through that week my baby happily went to school. The child we had when she was at home was completely different from the child we now had. When my baby melts down, she looks lost. She cries. She screams I hate you all. She wriggles around on the floor. She hits the other kids. She really becomes inconsolable until we step in. We structure her and she can settle. Sometimes it takes a little while and some imaginative thinking to help her settle. She will though, it just takes time.

A recent episode was watching her just try and make it through the day. I was having my own bad day. No one had written on the whiteboard what we were doing that day. My son and daughter were reading, all day, as they do. My husband was outside cleaning the BBQ. My daughter was lost. By 3pm I'd had enough. I picked up my whiteboard marker and wrote her a schedule. It involved a bath with Mummy's special bath bomb, making dinner with Mummy and helping Dad to wash the BBQ. It was really clear and structured. She went up and screamed. She picked up the marker and ticked all the activities and screamed 'There. They are all done. 'She started crawling around on the floor again complaining and crying until her sounds became like fingernails crawling on a blackboard to me.

Amazingly, she stood up. She went to the fridge and took out a red capsicum. She took a plastic bowl and cut the capsicum into chunks. My baby walked to my room and took the bath bomb. I said nothing, just watched. She went to the bathroom and called out to me to come and see the colour change of the water. She put herself in the bath. She had her capsicum sitting on the side of the bath. She stayed there for 45 minutes playing quietly. The heat of the bath, the moisture of the water, the structure of the day; I had given her support. Without being able to articulate how lost she was, she was begging for support. Without becoming angry, I was able to provide support. I applied my knowledge of Ayurveda and Vata imbalance to support my baby. A year ago, I would not have understood and would have been yelling at her. Awareness is the first stage of being able to modify lifestyle to support behavioural needs. It is not always easy but sometimes it works!

My whole family are also loving our nightly routines. Warmth is just splendid. I keep my space and air in check as much as I can by applying warmth. Space and air are cold. I love warmth. The kids know my routine. The coffee place knows my daily order:' Extra hot coffee. 'Extra hot is what helps to relieve every single piece of tension from my body. Standing in front of the fireplace is heaven. Going to sleep with two or three extra toasty wheat bags is just sensational. Summer, I love! Heat for me is just magnificent. I spend so much of my time watching and keeping things in check and the application of heat helps to let go.

Heat in food. Cooked meals. Salads and raw food are great in summer but for meals that are truly digestible, the application of heat to cook food makes it easier to process. Raw food is considered to be dry and cold. Textures can be so important to people with autism. Crunch, smooth, texture. Diet in autism is critical.

Recent research suggests the lifespan of people with autism is lower than neurotypicals. One of the reasons suggested for this reduced lifespan is diet. Many people with autism experience restrictions in eating. This goes beyond the yoga concept of attachment. The ideology in yoga of suffering is based on the concept that the way that we think affects our wellbeing. Some of the connections with yoga, nutrition and autism are related to attachment and avoidance. Yogic theory suggests attachment is about pleasure seeking. Attachment to foods that are considered pleasurable results in suffering through an inability to be flexible. This may result in fixed ideations and prevent alleviation of suffering in that area.

Yogic theory also suggests avoidance is a cause of suffering. My girl avoids textures. This has affected our family meal sessions with her refusal to eat meals with us at dinner times. Usually by dinner time I am already exhausted and now I know why. All the executive functioning and masking that I have been holding together means my resources are depleted. My husband, who has escaped the family home to go and teach a bunch of teenagers as a school teacher, is also exhausted from managing classes and different personalities all day. The only problem is, you cannot avoid meals.

I used to manage this really well when my girl was little. I would start with a drink in my hand about 3pm. Never before 3pm. The rule was drinking was only allowed at 3pm. Then by the time dinner time came around my senses weren't as heightened and I didn't really care that much. Otherwise, it would be meltdown frustration city. We thought she was just being stubborn. Now we know better and now I don't touch alcohol.

One of the unfortunate side effects of being a mum who melts down, and having a wife who melts down, is the amount of tension in the house. My husband would need to take care of the children's needs, including helping my girl eat, because I just couldn't cope. I would consider it a personal insult and my ability for control was often compromised. The other part of the puzzle was my girl's inconsistency. Sometimes she would eat and sometimes she wouldn't. I saw this as a slur on me and became super frustrated. Frustration and autism generally leads to meltdowns, not a calm family, all sitting around the table with the intention of spending some quality time together whilst discussing the day. It was tense in our household.

Food for some people is nourishing. Food for others is social. Food can be just a part of life or food can be torture. I consider myself fairly lucky. I understand some people who present with autism have huge control issues around food. I have worked with kids with extremely limiting diets. I am in awe of their parents' patience. Products on the market have been designed to help keep food items separated or colour coded. This is a real source of stress for some people with autism.

For me, food is about control. My girl wouldn't eat. Sometimes she would. I had no control. My boy would eat everything. My baby would eat everything. What was wrong with my girl? She must be acting in defiance. Wrong. She could not swallow the texture of the food, and my attachment to the way meal times were supposed to be, as well as my attachment to having parental control to make her eat her meal, was compromised. In addition, my girl's avoidance of food textures was not defiance, but to do with a sensory experience she could not handle. In the wisdom of the yoga philosophy, we both suffered - my girl through her behaviour of avoidance and me through my attachment to what constitutes a good happy meal and a well behaved and compliant daughter. Remember, by the end of the day my spoons were out; and I grew up in the *Brady Bunch* era when families happily sat and ate meals together.

Food is also about alleviating anxiety for me. Enter now the world of the eating disorder and autism. I am a perfectionist, of sorts. I have been taught to be. My mother when I was young would say to me, you are perfect. At this time, we had no idea I had autism and one of the characteristics of autism can be the interpretation of words in a very literal sense. So, I had to be perfect.

On the other hand, my father would tell me I was crap. Maybe in a few more inventive words than that though. One parent is confiding in me and telling me how good I am and the other is pretty much telling me how pathetic I am - and how fat I am, which means that, quite simply, I am dirty and unlovable.

Here comes the clincher. I have to pretend to be perfect. I have to act so no one will see the dirty little girl I really am. If they don't see me as perfect then they may realise I am just a fraud and leave me.

The method of perfection was simple. Get skinny. Skinny means no more dirty girl. Skinny means I can wear what I want and people won't leave me. Got it. The only thing is, getting skinny is hard. And the road to getting skinny meant that I had to do some pretty dirty and secretive behaviours. This negates now any perception that I might be perfect and helps to compound my father's words that I am literally nothing but a piece of dirt who is totally unlovable.

Treat that. How? Every single thing I just wrote is logical. It is, I hope, clearly written and structured. The only issue is that the logic is the logic of a neurodiverse child and the world of the neurotypical would not see things in the same light. So, treatment becomes based on the model of physical and biological intervention and bypasses any consideration that there may be a completely logical but different way of thinking about systems operating here.

There is more and more research into eating disorders and autism. It is needed. I began as a failed anorexic. I was diagnosed with bulimia. This was a very dirty and secretive way of being. Ew. Finally, when I summoned all my strength, I was graced with the label of anorexia. The only issue was that I was now so controlled in my anorexic behaviour that any deviation was to result in a huge upheaval of anxiety. My body was so emaciated that I had no energy. I lost all social connection and fell into a pit of deep depression that fluctuated for ten years. I also developed a very strong attachment to clean, so much so that my body would be scrubbed up to 20 times a day in the shower and the parquetry floor was swept in the same direction at least an even average of 10 times a day. These behaviours support the disorder of anorexia and help to alleviate the anxiety of autism. They all serve a function.

In Ayurveda, it is suggested not to target habits by removing the behaviour. To do so would simply result in anxiety or in the behaviour returning because there has been no scaffolding to support the space. Remember that earlier discussion of space and air? When there is a gap, it really needs to be filled. Instead, Ayurveda advocates to replace behaviours that cause suffering with something else, and gradually increase the balance until the habit naturally falls away. I tell you this works! I left hospital as a day patient at Royal Melbourne to study Psychology. Against all the recommendations from the hospital experts. I was considered defiant and told that if I left, I would not be welcomed back, and that I was too sick to leave. I left. I have never looked back and I have never had another hospital admission for an eating disorder. I simply replaced my behaviours that were not self-sustaining with another one - an obsession with the mind. Hello person with autism!

There are many reasons why a person with autism may develop anorexia, or any eating disorder. My trajectory to anorexia was paved perfectly by my parents. Stress related, anxiety induced stomachaches, then headaches, then an eating disorder was clearly paved by the emotional turmoil of living as an undiagnosed female with autism and the transition to menstruation and teenagehood.

Many people with autism experience food sensitivities. This may be through food textures, foods touching, sensory overstimulation or an inability to properly digest foods.

Autism is characterised by complications with social interaction. When this affects day to day functioning, it may lead to a reduction in quality of life. Often the transition from primary school to high school starts to unravel the peer support network and safety supports the child had in place in primary school. Now not only is there generally a wider network of different energies to navigate, there is also a change in routine, accompanied by a change in peers. Zucker, N (2015) conducted research on females with anorexia to explore the relationship between peer support and eating disorders. Zucker's (2015) report is eerily close to my own personal expression of an eating disorder as a method of controlling pain caused by changing responses in a social culture.

My darling baby experiences behavioural dysregulation. To put it bluntly, she is a fire cracker. We love her dearly but don't always manage her behaviour too well. Before we had the language of autism I struggled. I was told she had a highly strung personality.

I was told it was developmental and she will grow out of it. Nope. She has autism, with no strategies for emotional regulation because I, as her mother, have also not been taught strategies that are healthy for emotional regulation and her father is so burned out being the mother's carer that my baby has had to fend for herself, or, when it became way too much, just get an iPod shoved into her hand so we could all get a break.

It is suggested in yoga philosophy and in psychology that we have cellular memory and this may exist deep within the core of the nervous system. Is there a genetic component to an eating disorder? I will not debate that here. Just ponder for a moment and make up your own mind. Where I am going is in the observation of my baby. She has a mother who experiences emotional dysregulation. She has a mother who has very late diagnosed autism and a colourful history of mental health issues including anorexia. My baby sits at the dinner table with her family most nights. When the mother is strung out, the mother does not join them. The mother eats differently from the family. Hmm.

My baby may genetically, from a biological and epigenetic perspective, have a pre-disposition already to an eating disorder. Her environment may also support the development of an eating disorder due to the social learning theory's explanation of behavioural acquisition through observation and imitation. To put it bluntly, my baby may be a sitting duck. In addition is Moseley et al.'s (2020) exploration of unidentified emotions as a trait contributing to the development of anorexia for people with autism.

Alexithymia is a term to describe problems with emotional identification. This is a common trait experienced by people with autism. Emotional dysregulation is simply being unable to control or regulate emotions. The thing is, first you have to identify what they are. Ask me when I am in a meltdown what I am feeling and what my emotions are and I will rip your head off. Ask my baby what she is feeling and she will rip your head off. Or she won't be able to answer verbally. Food. Now this is a tool to be able to rid oneself of the stress of emotional dysregulation. For a person with autism who cannot control emotions, food is a method for keeping control and alleviating some of the anxiety of not being able to express what is going on.

Does this mean my baby will develop anorexia? Not if I can help it! As a family we are putting in strategies for behavioural regulation now that we understand she is not crazy nor is she a bad child. She simply has autism, and we are trying to help develop the language of emotional identification to reduce the overwhelming, flooding effect that happens in the inability to emotionally regulate. There is no way I would watch any of my children suffer the way I have without fighting for them, whether they know it or not.

There are many different reasons why an eating disorder may develop. In my book *Food Hurts - Healing Anorexia Nervosa and Bulimia with Yoga and Ayurveda* I provide a very real representation of what an eating disorder may look like from the perspective of the patient. It hurts. I also provide a section on how I dug my way out of that hole using yoga and Ayurveda. What I know now is that in my case the addiction of an eating disorder was simply symptomatic of a misunderstood young girl in pain with undiagnosed autism.

It is beginning to become common practice now to perform a partial diagnostic assessment to screen for autism at the onset of hospital admission for patients presenting with eating disorders. The New South Wales Health Plan for People with Eating Disorders for 2021-2025 provides an overview of the management strategy for patients who present with eating disorders. Early intervention for food avoidant behaviours, particularly for children who present with autism, provides best care outcomes. This demonstrates the beginning of recognition of a link between eating disorders and autism.

Newly emerging advocates such as Tony Attwood are discussing on an international scale the prevalence of eating disorders amongst people with autism. Professor Attwood suggests the statistics may be as high as 1 in 4 patients with an eating disorder also experiencing a comorbidity of autism. This means the treatment must be different. What I experienced as an inpatient for many years when my anorexia was at its peak resulted in further exacerbation of complex post-traumatic stress disorder and learnt methods to continue the illness. My experiences as a day patient with anorexia in a group setting were just horrific. I could not relate to my peers and am to this day surprised and shocked when I read the nurse reports that I was the group member with the lowest weight who did not try. I tried so hard and I thought I was the fattest.

There has to be another way. Professor Attwood, in his recent discussion with the Butterfly Foundation, a group to support carers of patients with eating disorders, advocated for client centred, individualised care. Professor Attwood speaks my language. Ayurveda is a model of health care based on a person centred, positive and empowering system of Indian medicine teaching skills in life. No two people are the same and subsequently treatment regimes should not be the same for everyone. Treatment is individualised and considered. This means there is an assessable outcome that can be monitored to evaluate the patient's progress. This also makes it expensive, and the individualistic approach does not satisfy the criteria of validated interventions according to Western medicine. This makes it hard.

The presentation of eating disorders can mask many things. Unfortunately, it can also exacerbate hidden illness or result in further complications. Obsessive compulsive disorder (OCD) is one such example. The underlying function of OCD is to alleviate suffering in the realm of painful or fearful thoughts. This results in behaviours that become addictive and controlling and if left untreated may begin to affect the quality of life. My son would bring his food up to his nose before he ate, every bite! Remember Kramer in *Seinfeld*? He did that too and there was a whole episode dedicated to this. Should these behaviours become extreme, then there is an issue.

When I scrubbed my body 20 times a day, my skin started to peel. This was an issue. There was no point telling me not to do it though. The action served a purpose and it settled my mind. Even today I have traits of OCD but they are not so crippling. I must exercise every morning. My mind is unsettled until I do. To challenge this is just too much and I'm just not prepared to go there. You know when I am truly unwell because I can't exercise. It's funny: even when I was in labour with the kids I would have to waddle around the streets, so strong were my thoughts that the fact that my body was about to go into exercise overdrive had simply no effect on my routine. This isn't affecting my quality of life though, and I can live with this.

My girl is exhibiting signs of OCD. Her little thing is order. Everything has to be in its place. If it is not, she knows! I even have to put the pen back the correct way or she writes me little letters to tell me how to do it. She has to touch a fingertip twice in the same way. Her toes have to roll in an even number of times. My girl calls these things her annoying little habits. Should they start to interfere with her daily functioning then I will need to intervene. In the meantime, these behaviours are exhibitors of the stress she feels and a method she has chosen to cope with anxiety in a way that works for her.

Once again, OCD is a signal that space and air in the body and mind may be in excess. Space and air like routine. OCD provides routine and structure. It provides a set way of doing things which allows the mind to focus on one thing. The issue according to yogic logic comes from the attachment of the behaviours. To not engage in the behaviours would result in suffering. Sometimes the engagement of the behaviours themselves will result in suffering and then this becomes an issue.

Yoga also talks about avoidance. To examine the function of the behaviour may be a method to find the core root of the issue. It may simply be to avoid feelings of fear or uncertainty. These feelings themselves may result in human suffering and block the ability to act from a happy place in this world.

Often in this world we operate within the one level. The psychological theory of Mazlow's hierarchy suggests that we have base needs. These base needs are essential for our survival and must be met first. They include food, shelter and warmth. (Please note the word warmth in relation to space and air.) It is impossible to move up to the next rung of Maazlow's ladder without first meeting the base needs. Yoga theory would look at the layers around us from the physical to the meta spiritual aspects. Most of us would operate from the level of the Annamaya Kosha. This is the yogic way of understanding Mazlow's hierarchy if you like. Most of us are concerned with the physical aspects that include the body, food and nourishment.

Often the physical layer, or sheath as it is also known, is taken for granted. Liken this concept to the layers of the onion. In order for eating disorders to begin to heal, there is more required than merely shoving food into someone's body. What is required is a more detailed understanding of how the middle core of the onion (the body) is also covered by multiple layers. These layers also have to be slowly understood for complete wellbeing. Concentrate on understanding the layers of the onion that make up the whole. It's a little bit like a spider's web - one move will pull the rest out of place. When life gets out of balance the layers get lost.

A person receiving care for an eating disorder primarily receives care with a particular focus on the lowest limb of Mazlow and the innermost sheath of the Annamaya Kosha. Personally, I have never been asked about the purpose of my anorexia. I could tell you in one sentence:' It helps me cope. 'The sad part is, I always could tell people that. I was just never asked. Understandably there is a medical emergency with an eating disorder that requires attention. This is not questioned. There are, however, different methods to begin to treat eating disorders, and as mentioned, there is growing research to suggest eating disorders and anorexia in particular have a direct correlation with autism.

Yoga has helped me immensely. It has kept me from literally going insane. For the first time I just felt like I was in my body and I wasn't competing. My mind, whilst not completely, was more clear, and the crap in my head was more settled. Not everyone is going to have this experience. Unfortunately in the world of yoga there have evolved many different styles and the public have become lost as to what yoga is. For me, yoga is about connection. I often find yoga off the mat in the words of my kids, in the smell of the rose, walking down the dirt road in the morning after a rainfall. My senses in these instances are calm. This is my yoga.

When I had to learn to eat again it was all about my breath. The anxiety was tremendous. Like many people with autism, I had this undying thought pattern that I was all in or I was all out. This meant my body was sometimes super duper stuffed - to the point of not being able to move - with green apples, or completely empty, with diet coke shoved down the hole to stop the hunger pains, drowned with multiple cigarettes. My sense of balance was shot by the autistic 'have tos 'and the amount of anxiety I just couldn't cope with feeling.

Another element of an eating disorder and autism is the accompaniment of other comorbidities. Unfortunately, as a middle-aged woman, late diagnosed, I had already gone through, shall we say, some tough times, and my husband and kids had to come along for the ride. Throw in complex post traumatic stress disorder and the whole thing gets blown way out of proportion.

Complex post traumatic stress disorder (CPTSD) is currently being debated as a possible underlying cause of borderline personality disorder (BPD). Professor Kulkarni of the Women's Mental Health Clinic and some groups that work with borderline personality disorder have discussed the possibility of CPTSD presenting as BPD. The suggestion is that the repeated trauma in a childhood may start to alter the chemicals and hormones, leading to an inability to properly regulate emotions. Where does autism fit in this? Many participants in autism Facebook forums discuss diagnosis of eating disorders, CPTSD and BPD prior to a diagnosis of autism. What does this mean for our wellbeing and hope for recovery?

One of the factors that often gets overlooked in a diagnosis of autism, when it is accompanied by psychosocial diagnosis, is the idea of deficiency. I will say this now and I will say it again: I am not broken. I merely have a different way of looking at the world. One of my special abilities, if you adhere to the notion that autistic people have some kind of superpower, is my ability to see situations from a bird's eye view. My observation is sharp. I have the ability to consider different objectives and make a snap evaluation from their point of perception very quickly. This infuriates my husband. He needs to speak. I have already summarised what he is discussing with me whilst he is in mid-sentence. The consequence is that he doesn't feel heard. We all need to feel heard, and when you are cut off mid-sentence, I am sure it feels just awful. I can also empathise with this position.

It makes it really difficult on all angles. For myself as a bird's eye view perceptive person and my husband as a person who has a slower tendency to think and assess situations. Remembering that autism is defined as a disorder that is associated with differences in communication, it becomes clear that communication can be confusing for all parties. It also poses difficulties when there are crossed wires of communication. Many times.

Humming in the ear when you are concentrating is awful. One of the side effects of stress is out of touch sensory experiences.

Uncannily, this is also a common finding in people with autism. There was a point not so long ago in my life when things were hectic. Now, I can cope with hectic. In fact, I am ever grateful to my attention deficit disorder (ADD) for giving me the ability to act on high voltage over a long period of time. Picture this: a person who is super passionate about something, has awesome abilities in research and the skill in navigating life from a bird's eye perspective and you have me! This can be unnerving for some people, but it has been a natural part of my lifetime operations, and to be quite frank, has kept me alive. In this sense I am grateful for my autism, but sometimes the body gives alerts. I have to be ready to hear. Enter tinnitus.

My children's diagnosis came out of the blue. Well, maybe not, but the realisation that they had autism was an out of the blue revelation. Before that, I just had no language to be able to explain what was going on. When you live with situations it is really easy to accept this as normal. Apparently, we were not living the norm. I knew I wasn't but I didn't realise it related to my children as well.

Managing their behaviours, navigating services for diagnosis, then navigating the National Disability Insurance Scheme (NDIS) system is really a full-time job. I also have myself to care for. Oh, and I teach and run a business, and throw in a Graduate Diploma of Psychological Science full time. I was coping. Then university stopped. I got lost. What on earth was I meant to do? Yes, all my assessing was up to date with teaching. My rosters at the Retreat were ready. My kids all had their appointments booked. I got lost in the silence. The silence began to fill the space with a hum. I still stand by a generator somewhere down in the paddocks around our home. I could hear it in the day and in the night. And it really bothered me.

My husband and my therapist both said it was tinnitus. No way. I went to the audiologist. I have perfect hearing. She said it was stress induced tinnitus. I wasn't accepting it. It had to be a generator. I went on a Retreat. Yes, you read that correctly. I took time out and went on a Yoga Retreat. In the middle of nowhere. The sound came too. How could a generator follow me to the Retreat? I honestly thought I was going mad. The worst part of my autism is that I become fixated very very quickly. I became fixated on the sound. I would go to bed searching for it. I would wake up in the night searching my hearing for that sound. As annoying as it was, once I heard the sound I could fixate on it. Hmm.

Looking after yourself on the spectrum is a full time job. Every hour of every day you need to analyse how you are going, how you are feeling, and what impact your behaviour is having on those around you. Now I also had to fit into my schedule the needs of three other children and hope to goodness my husband could cope.

Well, it turned out he couldn't. I watched him fall. Under the burden of all of this information I lost my crutch. He retreated into his own world. I asked him to take a break and get some time out. When I said this, I saw his shoulders relax with a huge exhale. I had read the situation correctly, and if I didn't act now, I would see him further retreat.

I felt frantic. The business was still ticking over and it gave me some joy. I was on university holidays, thank goodness, and all I had to do was manage the multitude of meltdowns that were being thrown my way the best I could. And there really were meltdowns. By now I had exhausted all of my resources and was frustrated with the whole system. I had tried to make appointments with carer supports but my details got lost in their system and appointment times were overlooked. Yes, there are supports for parents of young children. Yes, there are supports for carers, but most of these are during the day and inaccessible for the likes of my husband. And I sit on the fence with a foot in both camps - I have autism and I am the caregiver of three children with autism requiring fairly substantial intervention - the only issue is they don't look like it. Autism - the hidden disability.

I read about people with autism and noise cancelling headphones. I have used earplugs and I love them. It just kind of takes the edge off things and I can take a breath, but I can't eat with them in. I hear myself breathing. If I cook, I can't hear my food and I cook with my senses, so whilst they are good, they also have their unwanted side effects. Noise cancelling headphones are all the buzz. Literally. I bought this beautiful green pair. Green for calming. I kind of liked that! I'm calming my sense of hearing. I put them on. They are heavy. Woah. So heavy. I hear a buzz. This time it is not the generator but a high-pitched buzz, kind of like what I used to hear when I had hearing tests for grommets as a child. I hate it.

I have some wireless earbuds. These feel better in my ears and I really do like them. They are not heavy. I looked into some noise cancelling ones with a microphone. Perfect for when I take the kids shopping. Now, I don't know if I am alone here, but they are still sitting in the box. I am almost too scared to see how they work and whether I like them or not. It takes me a long time to try things.

I have this ideology that things need to be perfect. The other day I sat with my mother in a therapy appointment with my therapist. It was my therapist's idea that my mother might benefit from having the opportunity to learn about autism and consequently I might also benefit. Had my therapist not told me she would be retiring soon, I might have decided otherwise, but I completely trust this therapist and so I agreed. I will let you use your imagination as to how I approached that session. I masked to the absolute degree and a few days later I fell down, hard.

Anyway, I got through it and hopefully my children will benefit. My relationship with my mother was almost irreversibly damaged when she read all my diagnostic reports and disputed the diagnosis. That left me exposed and vulnerable. One thing my mother said during the therapy session, though, was of interest. She said that when I was young, she would tell me repeatedly that I was perfect. I wonder if a literal interpretation of that has somehow landed in my inner psyche, and I have this perception that everything has to be perfect.

If things are not perfect, I panic and blame myself. This is kind of just how it is. I am disassociated from that panic though. I feel the responses but my mind has this incredible, huge, impenetrable barrier that allows me to act clinically. I don't show the emotion, or even feel the emotion, if there is a crisis. I do, however, crash either the next day or a few days later. And I feel panic.

The sheer panic about whether these new noise cancelling ear buds will be perfect prevents me from opening them and trying them on. When I buy clothes, they sit in my cupboard for weeks on end in case they are not perfect. When we book holidays, I usually end up in a panic attack five or so minutes before we arrive in case it is not perfect. This is exhausting.

This perception of perfect is highly debilitating. I have prided myself on being perfect to the point where I feel I have become competent at all things but a master of none. My ADD gets in the way and the ability to settle and fully embrace gets side-tracked by the rabbit holes. Often, they are rabbit holes of survival. So yes, I act perfectly in a crisis. In fact, I am brilliant within a crisis. Then I crash. And I crash hard.

This ability to see things from a bird's eye view also helps with my parenting. The perception of perfect is also debilitating. I have to get the right things for them at the right time. I am a terrific advocate and concentrate really well to make sure their needs are met; however, I change my mind left right and centre after I analyse all the different options and this throws us into a spin.

I read a wonderful line in *Spectrum Women, Walking to the Beat of Autism* edited by Barb Cook and Dr Michelle Garnett. The editors invited autistic women to tell their story. ARtemisia in her contribution wrote about the idea that we are more than just autism, unless we are damaged from comorbidities such as post traumatic stress disorder (PTSD). I have been awarded a double-edged sword in this life: an ability to see things from the bird's eye perspective coupled with the inner longings of a broken and anxious inner child.

Recently enough was enough. I hit rock bottom. My kids needed me, or so I thought. I was out of spoons. I could not give them a hug at night because I couldn't get up off the couch. I had spent all day navigating their service providers, attending meetings for the children, doing my own counselling sessions, and I was out. Hit hard.

Service providers can be so well meaning. We are beginning to find our tribe and have some really really caring people who are reaching out. What becomes difficult is the added social pressure to be able to perform with these new people. They all understand autism, probably more than me, but I live it. Meetings wear me out. An hour is my limit and then I burn out and my inner voice is saying leave and my inner child is saying run away and hide - I can't take anymore. So I reached a stage of carer burnout. My husband also reached a stage of carer burnout. Whew.

Stand up please the parent who has the most experience in dealing with service providers, has watched their whole life the intricate social system to try and work out what is happening and who also happens to be a control freak. The answer would be me. When one parent goes down, the other has to step up. What happens when both parents go down? Life has to change. The spoons are all out and television and electronic devices start to get a really good work out. On this note, I take my hat off to single parents. I honestly don't know how you do it and I am in awe of you.

So now both of us have carer burnout. This isn't really depression. It is more like…emptiness. Yoga and Ayurveda might call it reaching a Tamasic state. This is a mental state where everything feels stale and the life force has been sucked right out of you. Getting off the couch is so bloody hard when in reality, you just need to put your feet down and stand up. There is no fire left though, because just for a bit, the fire has burned out.

I had been watching my husband like a hawk for some time now. I need him so he can help me. It's kind of a vicious circle. My mood is regulated by his mood presentations. It's not the healthiest way of being for either of us and I am working hard on that. Given that the diagnosis of autism is very new, and I am in my tender age of mid 40s, and include the fact that we have been operating like this together for over 20 years, we have a long way to go to adapt our relationship to autism. So, I need him to keep it together.

Sometimes people who don't have autism get frustrated. Sometimes my husband will say it's the autism when really, I know it isn't. Sometimes he sees the complex post traumatic stress disorder rear its scared little head and sometimes he sees the roar and terror of premenstrual dysphoric disorder lash out to tear out his throat. The poor man can't win. Now combine this with three lovely angels who have very very recently all been diagnosed with autism and you have a very complex and at times dysfunctional family.

Coupled with this, my husband is a teacher. Teaching is becoming more and more intricate. He has been teaching now for over 30 years. He is at work teaching all day. I am home because I work from home (or try to!). The kids come home. One has a meltdown. I have a meltdown. We all have a meltdown and it takes us a long time to all clap hands together. I watch my husband's face.

I listen to his words. Sometimes the pain behind the words comes out. Logically and intellectually, I can see. I can't always hear it though because I need to be in the right head space. He says one thing, I understand another. I say one thing, he understands it differently. But how can this be? I have been so clear and so logical in my thinking. I have been carefully clinical in my approach. What the hell happens?

The crunch came a few weeks ago. I asked my beloved husband to leave. I was watching, responding, and tiptoeing, and I just decided I couldn't live like this anymore. I emailed him a very carefully worded email. I was also autistically meticulous and broke down our finances so he could see that we could still operate together and he could go to university next year as he had hoped to pursue nursing. All was good. All was clear. I thought.

Bombshell. I wasn't sure why he reacted the way he did. I broke my husband. He had to leave work after reading my email. This man never cries. He rang me at 11am. I had sent the email at 8am. He told me he was looking for a place to live and a job. Woah and slow down. All I had said was maybe you should think about studying in Melbourne. Suddenly we were splitting up and he was looking at dividing things. But this is not what I meant. The man broke.

Now I knew what to do really well from here. I shut down. I became clinical. Autism eat your heart out. I am very well trained in suicide response and a very good clinician for youth work and welfare. I have both formalised studies and lots of experience. So, I ran a mental health safety check on my husband first. All good. He wouldn't come home but he was safe. He was stuck sitting in a carpark thanks to Covid but, thank God, he was safe. Next, I rang all the services I knew to get help. One of the service providers told him an option was to leave me. Ok, hold it together Sarah. Don't let your tears flow.

My husband came home. Six hours later. I love him. I am so sorry to have not had the skills to communicate properly to him. Sometimes they say a crisis becomes a turning point, if you can be aware. This was just another turning point in our lives.

My husband conceded that life was too much for him. He took the week off work. Sometimes I wonder how autistic he may be - I had to repeatedly tell him to stop working for the first day! He went to the doctor and was formally diagnosed with carer burnout. I had tried to stop this, I really had. I could see it.

This left me on my own without any informal support now. I arranged for him to have a therapy appointment and argued that irregular counselling is inefficient for long term support. He conceded. For the week, I was on tiptoes.

My turn. Someone once told me the universe will only give you what you can handle. Well then, I must be bloody strong because the universe appears to continue to be dishing it all out to me. That weekend was probably the biggest meltdown experience of our lives.

Covid. School. I don't think there needs to be much more said here. We decided, with the principal's support, to send our children to school. They cannot cope without structure and I am way too scattered at home to support them. Combine this with my husband having to continue teaching online and school being taught on computers, it was not a very productive approach for anyone. We could have coped with this; however, the instability was beginning to result in an increase in aggressive meltdowns, and all of the people with autism in our family were beginning to have meltdown interactions - if that is a thing!

School was really good. We had to force one child, but the other two loved it. Finally, they were back in a routine and they knew how to play the game. Even if it did look a little bit different and the game posts were a little bit more narrow than what they were used to. My husband had the week off work and he was starting to feel a little more like himself. He decided to play with the kids. I was in my happy place, studying. Finally I could get back to study and start to navigate some of these over looming assessments. Then bang. Meltdown.

My baby had accidentally broken one of my vases. She panicked. She ran screaming out of the house. I ran out. I thought something tragic had happened. I had gone from this blissful state, where I was completely immersed in an autistic hyper-focused way, to intense loud noises and screams. She ran out of the house. My husband just looked at me. Every time we tried to console her she ran away more, screaming these awful guttural screams. I let the dog out, thinking the dog would console her. The dog ran up the paddocks in the opposite direction. This went on for 20 minutes. We just left her.

My husband and I re-grouped. She wasn't calming down now and it had been about 40 minutes. Right. My concentration was out the window and I was so worried about her, and him. I jumped in my car and started up the driveway. My baby started running up the driveway just in front of me. She had thongs on and was still screaming. I was so worried she would trip on the big rocks in the driveway. I reached alongside her, wound down the window and yelled out 'I'm going to Grandma's. Want to come?' This child loves my mother.

She actually got in. We were getting worried she was going to run to the highway. Thank goodness. I locked the car doors from the inside. She was still screaming. She put on her seat belt. She actually put on her seat belt. I rang my mother and told her to meet me at a local hotel carpark. Her first response was to tell me she wasn't dressed. I didn't really give a damn at this stage. I might have snapped. I might not have. I have no idea. I just drove up the freeway. I steeled myself. Ten minutes in I put on the radio. I found some music. Usually, I listen to talk shows, which I find soothing. The music worked.

I heard this little voice from the back. 'Did I break your vase Mummy?' My baby was back. I stopped my tears. This wasn't the time. I pulled over and got in the back with her and just hugged her. I told her it was ok. I didn't care. Daddy didn't care. I rang my husband and she heard his voice. He told her he didn't care. I needed him to know she was safe. I needed to hear that he was safe.

I drove to the carpark and handed my baby girl to my mother. My beautiful baby girl. She was timid and drawn. Later, when I called, my mother had given her Panadol because my baby had a sore throat. I knew why she had the sore throat and told my mother to give her ice-cream. My poor baby.

I had something else to contend with. My boy. He had been having his own time out at Grandma's house. I had, in desperation, pulled the pin an hour early for him. He was not happy. He was upset that my baby had once again been put before his needs. This is how he saw it and I can see it from his perspective. He had shut down. Covid masks and hoodies are excellent for hiding. He was wearing both. And we were in the car.

I had deliberately chosen a carpark with a drive through coffee take out. I needed one. I asked my boy if he wanted a hot chocolate. He told me that he felt like I was buying him off. I understood that too. Maybe I was. I also wanted to get something warm, sweet and grounded in his body. Quickly. All of my Ayurveda knowledge tells me that nutrition is the core of health. My son was shutting down and rightly so. For years we have responded to his sister's needs as the priority because he seemed just fine. It wasn't until the paediatrician said to us that he was our priority that we started to understand the impact of his autism on his abilities.

Autism meltdowns can be a result of too much socialisation, too much masking or too much sensory input. There are multiple reasons for meltdowns. My Ayurvedic understanding tells me this is a Vata type issue I am dealing with and therefore to pacify, or reduce, the Vata I need sweet and I need it now. Hot chocolate is not really the sweet that ideally I would have chosen, but it was accessible and available and I had hoped he would take it quickly. Ayurveda teaches me that air and space needs fast grounding and heaviness and the milk, warmth and sweetness of the chocolate meets all these requirements.

He had his hot chocolate. I started to watch him re-emerge as well. The mask had to come off to drink. The hoodie I removed from his head. We drove home. As we drove he started to talk. For our family, driving is the best. I am present for the kids and I can't multi-task, or attempt to multi-task. This means I am all ears for them and I can hear them without the distractions of home.

He shared with me how he feels second best. He wants relationships but home can be tense. How the meltdowns affect him. My radar was up and I was listening for those themes of depression, anxiety, helplessness. I wasn't hearing it yet, but everything I read is about early intervention being paramount to avoid later additional diagnosis. At this stage I was grateful my son was able to speak with me.

Home again, my daughter decides she can't go to school. She shuts down. This is number three in the day. This is the day I had set aside to enjoy my hyper-focus special interest to study psychology. Nope. Out the window it is going. My daughter's meltdowns are different again. She becomes mute. She squeaks. She has this look about her that I can now read to say I am not coping please help. She had loved school the week before. She was super duper excited to be back and managed really well. The reality of lockdown and another week of different school was becoming an issue. It was school but it wasn't really school. It was different.

I am not proud to say I lost my cool. The tears from my daughter were squashed flat. My tension with my mother was still paramount in my mind, even if she didn't know it existed. I was worried about my son. I just couldn't do my daughter as well. I snapped and yelled. Suddenly every little thing out of place was too much. The bird was too loud. There was too much to do. My husband calls it barking orders. I felt out of control.

I grabbed my daughter by the hand and sat next to my bed. I also had a copy of the book *Camouflage: The Hidden Lives of Autistic Women* by Sarah Bargiela in my hand. I just opened the book at page 1 and we started reading together. Then we started giggling. We are both so autistic and we could see each other in the book. We started pointing out the behaviours that were because of autism, like the way I eat the same thing every day. The way my daughter collects things. The way we both get overloaded with sensation. This book was a godsend. My daughter went to bed and to school the next day.

Tuesdays and Thursdays are my yoga mornings. My husband has always said when I am not around things are calm and he manages the kids really well. Hmm. I had been in yoga and had just cried. The words of yogic wisdom hit my heart. I was so calm afterwards and walked into our home. The tension. I could feel it. My baby had experienced a meltdown because she did not eat off a red plate. My son had gone to school already. My husband looked worn out. I rang my son to say good morning and heard it in his voice. Meltdown. Oh God. I had my own plans that morning.

I told my son to wait at the bus stop, grabbed my daughter and went to pick him up. I was still in my pyjamas (let's pretend they were yoga clothes). He had on the mask and his head was down. He was tripping when he walked. He got in the car. His tears were trying so hard not to flow. Enter clinical supermom. I emailed his support teacher from last semester. She was just brilliant and contacted me before school hours immediately. She asked where we were. I will give you one guess. Yup: drive through hot chocolate time again. I really must find a better way.

I drove my girl to school. My baby was already at school. I watched her stand out amongst her peers. Proud, strong and full of energy. My son saw her too. We spoke to his school whilst we were sitting there and learned about the school's sensory rooms and quiet spaces. My son agreed to go to school, but to the quiet room first.

On the way, we spoke. We shared about how the family moves and flows with meltdowns. He said how hard it was for him. My tears were further squashed down. I made him a deal. I told him I was trying, really trying to get something happening for supports. I just asked him for time. I told him that if home was still the same in six months 'time I would talk to his dad and we could possibly agree to let him live with my husband's parents down in Melbourne. I broke then and cried a little. Whoops.

We run a Retreat Centre and for Covid reasons we were currently closed. I offered him the opportunity of a room at the Retreat for a week. Just on his own. The room is under our roof line but completely separate. My conditions were that he had to go to sleep at the correct time, no computer in the room and he had to join the family for meals. My son's relief was evident; he needed space.

We needed help and we needed help fast. I was tense. I was snapping at my husband. I didn't mean to, I just found I couldn't answer the little words anymore. It was too hard to say where to put the towels. What was for dinner was an impossible sentence to get out. I had reached my point. I also had my period. Gotcha! says the PMDD.

I told my husband I needed a break. He agreed and we contacted my mother. We both needed a break then and there but it was still two days until the weekend. She had something on. She was seeing my brothers for their daughter's special event. My heart broke. I really really needed help. I was always put second best and correctly or not, the CPTSD came up and I felt like I was once again second best. I needed to go. I booked a two night stay in a hotel ten minutes up the road for myself. I was leaving in two days, for two nights, with my husband's blessing.

I was burned out. Still I wanted my children. The pool was wonderful. So warm. So big. So empty. I rang my husband and asked him to bring the three kids for a swim. We agreed on a 60 minute time limit. They arrived. As soon as my baby spoke I knew I was badly burned out. I had no spoons at all. I hadn't even seen them for over 24 hours. I was losing my ability to properly parent. I was losing myself. Yes we swam. Yes there were two meltdowns and one hefty slip on the floor during that time period. Yes my husband looked tired. I could see it all. And I just couldn't do anything at all about it. I needed to recharge my batteries and get some spoons back. I needed to do this so I could save them. I, too, had carer burnout, and my husband and I were on our own.

So where to from here? Well, ever the planner, I have a plan. My intention is to access supports to prevent carer burnout in the future. We love our three children so very much. They are all so extremely different. This means all of their needs are different, and often I burn out from trying to be a super mum, preventing meltdowns and caring for the kids. This really means there is nothing left for my husband, and he is feeling the abandonment.

My therapist talks often in sessions with me about the perception I seem to have of saving people. This came up in the dreams I often had as a child where I used to have to save my brothers and my father. In my childhood I worked very hard to save my mother from my father. I was her confidante. I have never wanted my children to feel any pain, especially given how painful I have felt life to be so far. Unfortunately this is unrealistic. As my therapist said to me the other day, our children only need us really until they are about 6 or 8 years old. When they are young they are reliant on us. When they become older they need us for different reasons but they really can meet their own basic needs. So where does this leave me? I have been running around navigating service providers, working as their advocate for the National Disability Insurance Scheme (NDIS) and trying very very hard to prevent them from experiencing any suffering - so much so that I am suffering myself, and I have become a burned out carer and pretty tense wife.

I am attached to the idea that I need to save my children. Save them from what? They cannot be saved from pain. Pain and suffering are a natural part of growth, but I am well and truly fighting to be their saviour. When my mother won't play the way I want her to in order to help save my children, when activities I have meticulously planned do not go my way, or when service providers are not as forthcoming as I need them to be, I meltdown. I am attached to this image of having the perfect family.

If my therapist read that statement above she would probably jump up and down and hoot with glee. Yes, I wrote it. My family is an autistic family. No matter what I do or how hard I try to prevent meltdowns from happening they are going to happen and the sooner I realise this the better, for the sake of both myself and my family.

There is an expectation that autism can be fixed. No it can't be. There is also an expectation in my extended family that I am the broken one. The faker. The eccentric. The cold-hearted bitch. The crazy one. There may be another term here - autism. I have autism! My children have autism. Now to get on with being an autistic family.

One of the first challenges is to put in place the correct supports. As an older woman this is hard. Remember back to that line from ARtemisia - I already bring a lot of baggage and I am super intelligent in some ways. I have been studying psychology all my life really. It is just now that I am making it official by studying in a Graduate Diploma year at university. I have watched shows like the *Brady Bunch*. I read and reread Enid Blyton. I devoured books about the second world war and the hope of family in my early teens. I knew people. Kind of. I knew how to understand people if they played by the rules. When they didn't play the way I anticipated I had to become clinical so I could work out how to act the appropriate way. One of the best supervisors for this was my husband. He would be my debriefer and my confidant. It ended up wearing him out. It also meant that I was subject to some pretty hard words and I was already full of hurt. The day I asked him to leave, I meant it. But not leave me, just stop saying things about what I do because I already know.

I found a support coordinator (SC) to help me understand the NDIS and to navigate the world of disabilities. I was savvy enough with mental health care, but NDIS and disability are a different game and I had no rule book. It took me three goes to find a SC that knew my area and was available for support. This in itself can be traumatic. My SC told me to get a speech therapist assessment. If you'd asked me, I would have said that was a complete and utter waste of time. Look at all my credentials: I am obviously smart and have excellent communication skills.

I did as my SC requested. Oh my gosh. What a page turner. If you have been diagnosed autistic, I highly recommend a speech therapy assessment. It has helped my marriage. My speech therapist (ST) is excellent. She could read me, just like my therapist. This was confronting. I aced the written section of the assessment. Told you so. I could interpret sentences. I knew how to make meaning. Then she hit me hard. I could not communicate. What I was trying to say with my words was not what was being received by the listener. No way! I was certain she was incorrect. She pointed out the email I had written to my husband and said if she had received that she would have interpreted it to mean the marriage was over. That was not what I had meant. I had been clear and clinical. She also pointed out the issue with clinical - it was not always appropriate and could be misleading.

I felt like a baby learning to talk again. The ST shared with me her understandings of autism and communication. I had a high level of ability to interpret the written word. I had to learn strategies to learn how to make meaning when there were multiple layers. This included social settings and just living in a household. All the layers of meaning become lost in the interpretation amongst the overload of sensation and past trauma. She shared with me her analogy of growing up without the basic understanding of how to behave.

This made so much sense to both myself and my husband. It clarified why I could not take a break. It helped us to understand why Bali trips were fraught with details for every moment of the trip, and even if it was not recorded I had a daily sequence that would be followed. To deviate from this sequence caused anxiety. To have to keep to this sequence caused anxiety. This is a pattern that is not self-serving and becomes a cause of suffering.

The rule book also applies to micromanagement within the household. I recently read a Facebook post that if the carer died, who would know everything about their child? I am the same. I have my yellow book and I have my grey book. I have so much information stored in my head. Some of it is on google calendar. If I was ever to become unconscious there would be a big unknown mess to fix.

Micromanagement keeps things safe. I know where things are. The difficulty here is that the kids and my husband don't like the micromanagement and I am exhausted by it. To hold so much responsibility for four people in a household is too much. I have let go of parts of this management but it is hard. Our family has created a pattern through necessity. It helped to hold us together. Now it is time to break the barriers and still my husband will say to me, how can I help? Tell me how to do it. This is hard on both of us.

We also noticed I try to micromanage the children. In doing so I am inadvertently taking away their independence and resilience. Ironically, I have been trying to work out for years how to increase their resilience. My son will come home on the bus. As soon as he gets home I 'bark orders 'as my husband would say. I don't mean to. It is simply that there are a lot of things to do in a short space of time and I am worried they won't get done and that I will forget them.

My husband has been watching my son's face. Given my son have been gone from the home for over 8 hours and has had to manage his autism amongst his peers during that time, he is generally worn out by the time he gets home. I do give him a hug, but I am learning he needs a break. Giving him his own room at the Retreat has been a godsend for both him and me this week. I am learning to let go and he is growing up. My son rang me on Thursday after school to ask me to collect him from the end of the road - a ten-minute walk. He said he felt unwell and that he had tripped over again at school. I had my university class. I said no. It's the first time I haven't run to save him.

Any ability I had to concentrate on university had gone out the window until he came home. Just before his anticipated arrival time I texted him and told him to go to his room at the Retreat. To divert from the house. This was to help him re-centre and catch a breath. It worked. He walked past my window to his own room and gave me the thumbs up.

Another strategy we are using is a whiteboard. The 'barking orders 'are written on the whiteboard. It gets it all out of my head and gives my son the time and flexibility to do things in his own way. It is working. I can see his relief. And for the record, I hate the phrase 'barking orders'.

The ST has helped us as a family to realise what the 'barking orders' is really all about. It is an inability to properly communicate my needs to the family. When my needs are not communicated I am not receptive to their needs. Hence carer burnout.

My husband and I had a debriefing session with the ST. He has sat with me before with the therapist. It has usually followed a time of crisis and has allowed him the opportunity to debrief. This helped immensely. The ST also offered the same, with similar guidelines to the therapist. It was a one off session and neither therapist was offering couples therapy.

The ST did discuss couples therapy with us. It was her informed opinion that I did not have the skills for couples therapy and this may be more of a barrier. For therapy there needs to be a receptivity of communication. I am excellent at doing this one on one. With my husband though, I am trained to be on alert. I am sensitive to any comments, any looks, any phrases or examples that may indicate I am a bad person. Instead, the ST is working with us, and it is helping.

When my baby had her meltdown, my husband and I applied the tools from the ST. We wrote to each other. We did this in separate rooms and then showed each other what we had written. We were nowhere near each other. We had just spent the last hour talking and I was getting frustrated and he was getting frustrated. Voices were getting louder. I recognised this and put my hand up. This was time to stop. When we read what we had both written we realised we were saying the same thing but a different way. We were unable to verbally find the words to express what we wanted and the written word helped to clarify meaning.

My mother would write. She would write love letters to us as kids. She would write damning letters to us as kids. More recently she wrote to me saying I had destroyed Christmas with her children and my autism diagnosis was not real. (She has since retracted that last part, but the damage at the moment has been done for me.) To have my husband and me write was a trigger, but it is working, and I have faith that my husband will not do me harm intentionally. He has our best interests at heart and he is also a very talented writer.

I would often say to our family members that I cannot hear them. I have exceptional hearing for my age. I just could not hear their words though. My husband also has a lovely sounding voice with a very low tone. I find it very soothing. If my mind is busy, I can't hear him. It is more than that though, I can't process what he is saying. This adds to our confusion and frustration as a family. My girl's speech is so quiet I strain to hear what she is saying when I am sitting next to her. So does my husband. Unfortunately she will give up most of the time in frustration. We are still working on this.

Our session with the ST was enlightening. Not only do I have an unwritten rulebook, am very good at interpreting the written word and not so hot on writing or verbal communication, I also have to learn skills now in letting it go. To learn to sit with the anxiety and start to give my husband a voice. His voice is worthy and I am willing to listen. Both my husband and myself look forward to our next session with the ST and are excited and willing to implement what is to come next.

I continue sessions weekly with my therapist. She is retiring, and even writing this makes me cry. At least now I am crying. I think I was so shocked that I have moved through a grieving process and made plans and strategised for how to stay connected. I understand the therapeutic relationship. I don't know though how I will ever let her go. No one has been able to touch me the way she has. She has given pure hope where there was none. With her wisdom and experience she saw through the clouds and could read the situation. She has not only helped me but also our children. Recently one of my older friends said to me she is grateful for my diagnosis. Her son has also been diagnosed with autism and I am sharing my knowledge and resources. My therapist has not only touched me, but she has touched many many more people than she will ever know. I hope I write this well because I am sitting here writing this with tears streaming down my eyes and this is not clinical at all.

My therapist is my weekly go to. Together we have worked through depression, PMDD and autism. A diagnosis of autism can be shocking. I have moved through anger: why didn't anyone else pick it up? I have moved through grief: I am so old; I have had a life wasted; it is not fair. I have moved to needing to fix and change. Finally I am moving to acceptance. I am out and proud. I just can't mask anymore and I don't want to. Anyone who doesn't agree that I have autism can go jump. I do. I know I do. My therapist, thank you.

There is trauma there in my life. It stems way way way back down deeply into my core. I have tried so many different counselling techniques with so many therapists. My poor body has been so pumped full of medications and I would be listed at the moment as treatment resistant. So I need to find another way.

My therapist is trained in many therapies, but not Eye Movement Desensitisation and Reprocessing (EMDR). Given my history of trauma and my struggles with PMDD, my therapist suggested to me a specialist clinic in Melbourne. Again I am grateful to her for her insight and knowledge here. Another amazing person is now working alongside me: the GP I am seeing is incredible. I understand I am a very complex case. I present as a late diagnosed autistic woman with a luggage of comorbidities. Some are resultant of a late diagnosis and others are from the trauma of growing up in a dysfunctional family as a child. It really doesn't matter what the reasons or labels are, what does matter is how to treat it. This really is one of the benefits of labels. These disorders need to be treated differently. (I hate the term disorder too. We will take it to mean deviating from the norm and causing pain and suffering shall we?)

The GP and I have been working together for about a year now. We have trialled many medications for PMDD. It is a bugger to treat and it is almost impossible for me to handle sensation overload when the PMDD cycle comes around. My GP has shown care and compassion above and beyond my expectations. She is patient and answers all my questions and I am very grateful for her support. She takes a holistic family approach which is needed when there are four people in a home with autism.

My GP recognised there are three distinct layers of complications within my presentation. She referred me, at my request, for Eye Movement Desensitisation and Reprocessing (EMDR). This has not been comfortable for me. It has taken me two therapists to find one I like and trust.

The EMDR therapist is incredible. She is also trained in autism. I hate sessions with her. Well not really; but they are not comfortable. I don't know what she is doing. I also don't want to know. I understand cognitive behavioural therapy (CBT). I used this, or a version of this, to start eating again. I also understand other forms of therapy like schema therapy and have researched most of them except for EMDR. For a micromanager control freak this is a really good fit. Except it hurts. A memory is brought to the surface and together we work to process it using tapping. I prefer the tapping to the eye movement. The eye movement makes me feel a little bit dizzy.

Sometimes I cry. Most of the time it takes me until at least mid-session to feel anything at all. I am so well trained in autism that I am used to squashing the tears, just like when I had to get my baby to safety. The hardest thing, though, is that the onset of perimenopause is reducing the ability I once had to hold it together. Sometimes I just cry now and I am not sure if it is the floodgates of reconnecting strongly with my yoga practice again or the effects of EMDR. Either way, it is a not so comfortable relief.

Emotions are so embedded it can take some time to realise how they play out in the present moment. The incident of asking my mother to look after the children because I needed to get away with my husband is one such example. She had no idea I was burned out. I refuse to share anything personal with her, for my own self-protection. All communication of this incident is a relay between my mother and my husband. Neither of them realise how deeply hurt I am by the perception of abandonment and associated lack of safety. This is a theme that is coming up again and again in EMDR. Slowly, with the help of the EMDR therapist, I am learning to process it. I am so grateful for her knowledge and wisdom about autism and her willingness to sit and hold my hand. She recently promised me that she will not leave me if I am upset after a session. Thank goodness. So I continue with weekly EMDR to help develop the skills to manage my life. A life that just so happens to include autism.

Part of managing autism is also letting go. I have an SC who does her best with me. I am challenging. Hold tight, we can do this. I get really drained after appointments and most appointments with allied healthcare providers are an hour. I can manage this. Maybe I am even trained for this. I think back to the years of service provision I have had in my time with anorexia and every professional was an hour in duration. The same does not apply to support coordinators or support workers and I find this difficult to manage.

I contacted one service provider who suggested having a support worker for all four of the people with autism in our home.

This was one each, not one for all. I asked this service if they understood autism. Having that many people in our home all at once would send me into a constant meltdown. Imagine trying to let go of micromanaging that many people! Imagine the sensory overload of having that many people in the house all at once. I politely, or maybe not so politely, said no thank you.

My children and I are regarded as Complex. This means, apparently, that there are many of us living within the same household. I am very grateful to have had this explained to me as it felt really rotten to have a label of Complex on my head, especially in reference to my family. This means that we are able to access support services as all of our disabilities are lifelong and are not going to go away. I have heard from some people that they have been asked to get a current diagnosis if they have been diagnosed as a child and I laugh out loud. Autism in my mind is not something that goes away. It is not to be cured. It is something I am proud of, proud of my ability to think differently from the mainstream. It is just living in and understanding the mainstream that can be the challenge.

Say the word autism in a diagnosis and it is immediately recommended that you access three service providers, namely a psychologist, an occupational therapist and a speech therapist. I understand the purpose and intention of psychology. There is a process to go through when understanding the autism diagnosis and oftentimes anxiety is a hidden, or sometimes not so hidden, by-product of autism.

I had no understanding of speech therapy prior to my interactions with the ST. In fact, I was standoffish. Now I understand the importance of social communication skills. Having spent three years coaching my girl in social skills I really understand how important this is.

I had no prior understanding of occupational therapy prior to my diagnosis of autism. All I thought was that it was a service for old people or for work recovery. Overload! I sought out my own OT. I clearly asked for a diagnostic. My children had been assessed by a children's OT and I reached out to an adult service. What a difference. A benefit of autism is having a sixth sense. Some people have suggested extrasensory perception (ESP) or even telepathy. Whatever you call it, I have learned to listen to my gut feeling. And then I analyse it to death as I chew my husband's ear off. This adult OT just didn't feel right. Firstly, on the day of the appointment the therapist was apparently too unwell to travel out to me. Secondly, when we tried to connect online her camera wouldn't work. She was very good at asking questions and I was left stripped and bare with a dooming realisation of my own quality of life. I was in tears and fell down with depression for the few days that followed.

A week later I contacted the service and asked what was happening. Apparently, we had made another appointment at the end of the session. I had no recollection. Just a feeling of being stripped bare. It just didn't feel right. I was told it would take ten appointments for a proper assessment. I had witnessed in the meantime the excellent service from the children's OT and read their reports, which had detailed information gathered within a one hour consultation. I wasn't buying it. Another service provider who was taking advantage of the system.

I approached the children's OT and asked for an assessment for myself. They agreed and it was gold. Not only was it clear on where I was struggling, it validated what I had been experiencing for years. I was not crazy. I simply had autism. The OT went one step further and amalgamated all of our sensory profiles into one document. Now we had something concrete to help us learn how to manage the four people diagnosed with autism and we could see how our own individual sensory profiles affected the other family members. Gold.

I sat with this incredible Occupational Therapist a few months back and she did a sensory profile assessment with me. Oh my gosh. What a revelation! I had no idea I was so triggered by the sensory stimulations around me. I just thought the ticking clock driving me nuts, or the bright neon lights giving me a headache, was because I was a pain in the neck and highly particular. I had no idea these were all under the umbrella of autism.

I also had no prior knowledge of what the term 'executive functioning' was. My first SC was amazing with helping me understand that our home is not dysfunctional just because I am wound up so tight. She helped me understand that when you have sensory overload managing things can be hard. This can affect appointment scheduling, answering a phone and sometimes just getting out of bed. These are all things that affect day-to-day functioning and living life as an autistic person; navigating social responsibilities and trying to perform daily tasks can just get too much.

Having things like regular weekly appointments at the same time is golden. The only way I can keep up with three children and myself is to have those regular appointments. This really helps to reduce the anxiety and that unknown fear factor, which in Ayurvedic terms we would call Vata imbalance, or air and space elements in excess.

My family and I live in a rural area. Waiting lists are long. I have been around the industry long enough to know just how hard it is to get people that are available, let alone are a good match. In the past I have had my girl connected with two psychologists. Neither was a good fit. This means that we are back to the waiting lists again, and when all the literature and research specifies early intervention this is really hard for a micromanager who needs to protect her children to comprehend. So again I am not really sure how a SC will fit with our family, but I am willing to give it a go and support it as much as I can.

Being a small family with no informal support can also be tough. In university we looked at the concept of grandparenting. Our families have not had the kind of support that many other families do. There is no judgement here. It is just what it is. Navigating three children around for three appointments each is a full-time job. Include my appointments and I am fully booked. The things that calm me get side stepped to provide early intervention support for the children. What we are managing as a family right now is beyond what is sustainable. I hope a SC for the children may start to alleviate some of this pressure.

My diagnosis of autism has been a long time coming. It has been fraught with pain and suffering. It has been immersed in a perception of 'should' and 'have tos'. These rules are starting to become less poignant. It hurts. It feels uncomfortable. It feels right. I love you, my beloved autistic and neurotypical family.

Epilogue - New Year 2022

Putting it frankly, 2021 was an exhausting year. I had three children diagnosed with autism in early April. This was the result of a huge amount of research that I had been actively engaged in as the result of my own late diagnosis in November 2020. By July I had hit exhaustion point. I now know this as autism burnout.

I was also really concerned about the effect all of this was having on my husband. I could see he wasn't coping so well. The tangled web of supporting me in my role as mother and advocate for three children was huge. Helping me manage my disabilities was just another drain on already taxed resources.

I went back to my old behaviours and once again pressed play on a broken tape recorder. I reached out to family - this time, the other side of the family. I called them for support. The initial response was disbelief. What were they meant to do? We just let the kids watch too much telly. I begged them to help and they agreed to come for a visit. I called the sibling. It was the first time we had spoken in years, but I was so worried about my husband and trying to get him support that I swallowed any sense of pride I had left. The sibling agreed to contact my husband. She never did.

So began a tirade of misunderstanding and non-acceptance. We sat with the parents around the dinner table. "Utter rubbish" is the diagnosis of autism, we were told. The kids were good kids. There was nothing wrong with them. If they had autism then so did the parents. All my life I had been trained to try and reason. I really tried, and so did my husband.

We offered to share with them all the children's assessment reports from three different professionals. They chose not to read them. We tried to share with them how autism affected the children and us. I was told that they lived too far away and it was for our own family to deal with. I was broken though, and so was my husband. I did something unusual. I asked for help to clean my pantry. For me to ask for this support was pretty indicative of just how low I was. My kitchen was my safe space, but in the attempt to be a good mother and run the kids to a bucketload of appointments my safe space had turned into chaos. The pantry was cleaned and they went home. Duty done. For the time being, all was safe in our world and I thought I had support.

We had no contact for months. This isn't surprising. It is just the way that family operated with ours. I had already had support - the pantry, and nothing else was forthcoming. Christmas was approaching. I was learning to hate Christmas. When I was a child it was a magical time - we met with my cousins and extended family and there was food galore. Growing up Catholic helped because of the anticipation of something special. Since my own family had chosen to disown me, Christmas was becoming a point of pain. A reminder that I was different and dirty. I was alone within my own immediate family, and I was considered to be the problem.

So I did what any other autistic person would do. I planned. I love planning. I also love research. I can spend hours looking at hotels, investigating and finding the right hotel. I proposed to my husband that we stay in a hotel for two nights over Christmas, and Santa comes Christmas Day. The criteria for the hotel was to include a swimming pool and two bedrooms. He agreed, and I booked a place where I had stayed before. Amazing!

I also proposed that we go to his parents two days before Christmas, and spend a few days with them before heading to the city. He agreed. I was again pressing play on the tape recorder to be a good girl, with family around us. He also agreed.

Finally, I suggested we go a few days earlier again and stay at their holiday house by ourselves, without any of our children. Just a couple of nights alone. Now to this, he agreed with bells on! We had been waiting for the opportunity to have a break together. I had dreamt of being snuggled in his arms doing nothing but being together for a few months now. This is how I had got through the tough parts of the year. All done. All settled. All agreed with everyone. Yahoo!

By now I had come to recognise my triggers, and I was working really hard to avoid meltdowns. Most of my meltdowns were a result of overstimulation and feeling overwhelmed. I was practising yoga regularly. I was getting good amounts of sleep. My diet, though somewhat restricted, was very clean and natural. I was also working with a therapist focusing on Eye Movement Desensitisation and Reprocessing (EMDR) to heal past traumas and we were really moving forward together. My main therapist was retiring at the end of the year and I was going to miss her immensely, but I was coping.

We left for our holiday in great spirits! The drive down was fun. My kids are fun. My husband is fun. It was Christmas and this was going to be a great year, finally.

The year before we had felt the same way. I had pressed play on the same old tape and we had prepared to spend the day with my husband's parents and his sibling's family. We arrived the day before, taking two cars so I could leave a day earlier and open the Retreat for summer. Less than ten minutes away from our location, my husband rang me from his car. He told me to drive to the nearby park. I was told the sibling would not be joining us for Christmas Day because the partner was still upset by an argument a year ago. What? The kids were expecting cousins. I was honestly shocked. History was repeating and I was the cause. Needless to say I sank into depression. Dirty one that I was.

The argument, a year before that, resulted from me becoming upset when my husband's sibling stayed in my bed when we were on holiday without us knowing. The mother-in-law had invited the sibling to come with her two children to stay whilst my husband and I took a break together. The mother-in-law then sat on my bed when we returned and lied to my face, saying the sibling had just turned up. I had melted down. Someone was in my private safe space. I had tried to talk. Tried to reason. Finally, six months later, the sibling had invited the kids to the cousin's birthday. Yippee! My children had family again! My own family had long since turned their backs on me and my children had no contact any more with their cousins on that side of the family.

The day before I was working at the Retreat. I had just finished doing three massages and had a missed call from the sibling. She left a message saying that because of me my husband was unwelcome in her home. The message was just awful. I went in shaking and asked my husband what was going on. She had said nothing to him. I tried calling. He tried calling. She wouldn't answer. It took her about six months to answer and that Christmas was going to be the first time together since then, so I was already on edge. Unfortunately we had to tell our children. They were all distraught. Again, that Christmas we had to tell the children that they would not see their cousins, changing what we had planned.

For autistic children this is not good. Routine and structure is what holds together the fabric of daily living. We had to deal with the meltdowns and fall outs of both occasions. So this Christmas I was super pro-active to make sure nothing was going to harm the children this year.

So in high spirits we dropped the children off at the parents' home and bid farewell. Alone time together, just the two of us - finally. Except I was suffering from PMDD. This makes me especially anxious and I was fluctuating between anxiety and tears. I was doing my very best to control my moods and made sure I was getting extra rest and conceded to watching movies.

The children rang. My youngest daughter loves Whatsapp and did a live call. She asked me to say hello to the sibling's children. Apparently they were also staying over. Now, I have absolutely nothing against these children. In fact I don't even know them. I do know, however, that my children just love them. I also know that my three children have autism and my son spends most of his time alone in his room. I dealt with the knowledge that the cousins were there.

On our return, our youngest daughter went into a meltdown as soon as she saw us. Oh my gosh. The mother-in-law said multiple times that my daughter didn't act like that when she was looking after them. Of course not. The child has autism. Surrounded by people, with late nights for two days and a diet of highly processed foods, is going to cause a meltdown when the people she feels safe with return. I just nodded and smiled but I did begin to doubt myself. I forgot all the therapists' reports that had verified that this child did indeed have autism and ADHD and required support with emotional regulation.

So I coped. I smiled at the right time. I said for the twenty-seventh time how good the cooking was. I was polite to the father-in-law. The sibling came over. I had broken my computer on the way down and had to buy a new one on my break with my husband. I handled the sibling's visits with self-regulation strategies designing my new computer. I did well. The sibling and her children went home. They were to come back the next day to open presents.

I was super prepared the next day. I got up early and did my yoga class. My mother-in-law had presented me with a huge plate of pasta and seafood the day before. I had freaked. I don't eat pasta. My children had seen it and eaten it when she wasn't looking. I wasn't doing that again. I told my mother-in-law I had put on a lot of weight due to medications and really just wanted vegetables please. I couldn't mentally cope with cheesy, heavy foods. I also tried to explain that I was to be admitted to hospital in late January to help me with the PMDD and autism and with strategies to help me look after the children. She changed the subject. I spoke to a blank wall.

We had a great day! Presents were exchanged. My children were happy. The sibling and the children came. Again, I was cautious but coping. My husband left to go and buy batteries for my daughter's gift and I stayed at the parents' house. I wasn't comfortable but I did it. That afternoon, as they were leaving, the youngest of the sibling's children asked to stay the night again. It was all being arranged and I was watching. I spoke up. I suggested no. We were leaving to go to the hotel the next day and I could foresee our children being exhausted from another late night again and having meltdowns. My mother-in-law's response was: he wants to stay, what can we do? I tried to explain autism to her. I also knew that my mother-in-law had said the child had cried all night during the nights he stayed and wanted to go home. The father-in-law was tired because he had sat with him during these nights. It was decided instead that the sibling and her children would return the next day before we left at 9.30am for breakfast.

Not good. I spoke with my husband. I told him that I get anxious when packing. I get interference from the parents, who comment on things, and I end up, usually, in a meltdown, and then suffer guilt for days after because I become flustered and overwhelmed. With the addition of the sibling I wasn't sure how I would cope. He understood. We put in really clear strategies. I was to go for my walk as soon as I woke up, to help me regulate myself.

He would pack. Then we would have a lovely breakfast and leave by 9.30am.

The next day came. Everything went to plan. We were a great team, my husband and me. The sibling came in. My husband was at the car putting in the last of the bags. Three of the children were sitting at the table spread with deli platters and toasted cheese sandwiches, waiting to eat. I said hello to the sibling. She ignored me. My mother-in-law asked if she was going to say hello.

I was not prepared for what happened next. I had not strategised. She spun around with a loud no. Looking directly at me, she asked why I had not allowed her child to sleep over the night before. She said he had been crying all night and I had upset him. Simple: I told her our children had autism and they needed sleep. They had been in bed asleep by 7pm the night before. I thought this was sufficient.

She started yelling. I got flustered. She wanted a real response. I tried to explain that our children get overstimulated and this causes meltdowns, and we were trying to have a lovely family holiday. She kept going. The mother-in-law stood beside her. I asked the sibling to talk further outside, away from the children. She refused and kept yelling. Why on earth I didn't just leave, I don't know. I just couldn't. The father-in-law came in and the three stood in front of me. I started shaking and screaming to my husband that they were attacking me. I showed them I was shaking. The sibling kept yelling. The mother-in-law spoke. The father-in-law spoke. I couldn't take it all in. My husband wasn't there and my children were watching.

I snapped. I needed to go. Now. But I was shaking so much I couldn't think. I couldn't find my new computer charger. My hands were refusing to co-operate and the children were crying. Oh my gosh. I yelled. I have no idea what I said. Every piece of hurt came up and out. I had lost control, like a frightened little rabbit caught in an unexpected headlight turning into a vicious fox for self-protection. Not one of them understood autism. My husband came in. Finally I found my computer cord and escaped their house.

I walked out and saw five children huddled together on the front lawn. My heart just broke. I am so sorry, children, I am so sorry. My youngest daughter was screaming, with tears rolling down her face. I yelled at my father-in-law to hug his grandchild. I had no reserves left. I pleaded. He turned and walked back inside.

We got in the car and left. All four of us autistic people in the car were crying. My husband stared straight ahead, just driving. I wanted to rip my hair out. I wanted to slap my face. My children were still crying. I wanted to run away. How did this happen? What had gone so wrong?

We pulled over half an hour up the road, at a local shopping centre. I tried to be composed but I just couldn't hold it. This was Christmas Eve. We went into a café and I asked my husband to get three hot chocolates for the children and a chai for me. They had no chai. I had given up coffee three weeks ago so I went without. I wanted the sweet warmth to calm the children. My son refused to talk. His meltdown was strong. He refused to drink. My heart broke further. My youngest daughter, razor sharp that she is, told me what had happened. She took my husband and me through the incident piece by piece. I was provoked. I was a sitting duck in a lions' den.

Worse was to come. My husband, in the panic to escape, had forgotten his toiletry bag with his shaving equipment. We just looked at each other. I suggested that he go back to get it. I walked out of the café to another one. I needed a break. I ordered a take away chai from another café. When I returned, my husband said he was going back. I was on my own in a shopping centre with three kids in meltdown.

On his return he gave me the news. I was disowned. There was no such thing as autism and I was using this as an excuse for bad behaviour. I had been the instigator of bad behaviour in my family of origin and they could no longer put up with me. I was out of the family.

A rabid dog. For over 20 years I had made lots of effort. I had smiled and tried to be good. Our values, however, are not the same. They care about money. Their measure of success is in wealth. Love is in building gardens not in providing emotional support or care. The very fact that I had yelled was unforgivable, forever.

The feedback from the final meeting that day between my husband's family and my husband was twisted. I had decided the children were not to go to the sibling's home, the message from years ago conveniently forgotten. I am too hard to be around, with too many rules. What rules? I still can't work this one out. My rules are about me. I am not allowed rules at their house except for my morning walks. I don't even get to control what I eat. My attempt to try and get support, by sharing that I was going to hospital, was my own problem and they didn't even ask me about it. I do wonder who they think is going to look after our children when I am admitted, and what actually constitutes family support in their minds, but I'll let it go.

There are so many more things that could be written here, but I have learned one thing. It all comes down to perspective. My values against theirs. My expression of love against theirs. My diagnosis of autism and desperate need for acceptance, their unwillingness to accept that I am anything but a bad person. For me, the final straw was when my father-in-law walked away from my daughter. My mission now is to support my children from denial and prevent them from feeling the pain I have suffered. And my love, my husband, my deepest sympathy and respect goes to you. We share the same values. For his family of origin success is measured by wealth; for us, success is measured by the relationships and love between our children. I continue to teach them the goodness of humanity, but now they are witnesses to the events that unfolded. I had hoped to protect them from this.

We came together as a family once again and drove to the hotel. We all tried so hard to put it behind us. My gosh, I struggled. But I wasn't giving in. What else was I supposed to do? I sat in the spa on Christmas Day and read a book. It was about a lady who had experienced trauma, and her realisation that her coping strategies were regarded as odd in the eyes of society. The book was therapeutic. The reading was therapeutic. The water was warm. I worked hard on healing.

Melbourne during Covid was hard. The pool required a check point every time we used it. The cafés were busy. The restaurants were noisy. We learned so much about ourselves as a family that Christmas.

We learned that sharing what our plans are for the day is essential for self-regulation. Changes in that routine will lead to a meltdown. Too much choice on menus will lead to meltdowns. Spaces that have lots of people and loud music are going to lead to a meltdown.

So what does a meltdown look like? Panic on a child's face walking into a busy space. Grabbing my arm for support. Tripping over feet. Not being able to talk, not by choice but by mutism. Aggressive speech and behaviour, which looks like bad behaviour. Retreating for hours before climbing into my arms for hugs and reassurance. Constant talking about the same thing over and over. Stimming and tics. Wearing tracksuit pants on 38 degree days and refusing to take them off. Finally finding a place to sit and then needing to go to the toilet. And then needing to go again ten minutes later. Needing constant reminders to attend to basic hygiene. These may sound simple, but unless you are around someone with autism and seeing the panic, you really can't know just how hard it is for the person and the carer.

I also learned that I wanted to go home. I cancelled the extra night at the hotel. The children cried. They wanted to stay. Again I had to cope with meltdowns, but I needed desperately to go home to my safe space in my room in my bed. The bed that had been violated through ignorance and lies years before. Coming home was one of the best decisions I had made the whole trip. I was where I belonged.

I reached out. I asked for help from our family support worker and she came the next day. I couldn't make decisions for two days. I would just cry. I realised I was actually pretty traumatised and reliving what had happened. My youngest daughter also kept talking about it in various ways.

I reached out to Facebook sites. I contacted my publisher and asked for extra time to write this chapter. I contacted a friend. I found that the more I talked, the more I understood the ignorance that people have about hidden disabilities. I also understood that mental illness and disabilities are still not accepted in so many ways. I don't blame the ignorance of my husband's family. I probably looked like a psycho. But I am saddened that I was provoked by years of unsaid miscommunications and that I take the brunt of the punishment.

I hope one day my husband's family tries to understand autism in an attempt to really know our children, but I don't hold my breath. It is easier to victim blame me and stay in a state of ignorance. And when my father-in-law says there's no such thing as autism, and if there is I have autism too, then I accept that it really is a lost cause.

And going back to my cassette tape analogy, that play button, I have broken it. I will never press play and repeat the same mistakes with them again. I am stronger than that.

Letter from the heart of an autistic person diagnosed with ADHD, PMDD, and an eating disorder

Please see me. The core of me. Look behind the layers of clothing, the layers of blubber covering my body. Look beyond the bloated belly, the confusing behaviour. See me.

Be thin. Get skinny. Fat equals bad. The thinner you are the better. To be fat makes you unlovable.

So I get thin. I get even better than thin but I am still not good enough.

And I can't get out. The rules become too tight and I am trapped.

And you don't help me. You make things worse. The two of you together, you feed off me. I am your scapegoat, fat, dirty me.

You won't let me go. I don't understand your games. You bring in others, your own children, and cut me further down. Down, down, down spat.

One day, one of you goes. For good.

But the other holds on. Oh you hurt. You fight me. The good times confuse me. The bad times run deep.

I am empty.

Then you see me. And I see you. Years later with our children together I see them. I feel their pain. I hold them. I fight. For them. For acceptance. For love.

And finally I see me. For who I am. I am good enough. I hold me now.

Appendix

Resources We Designed in our Family

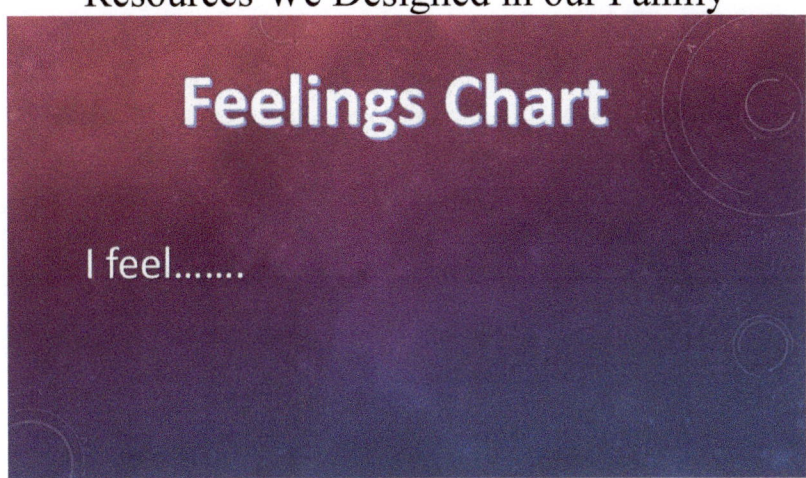

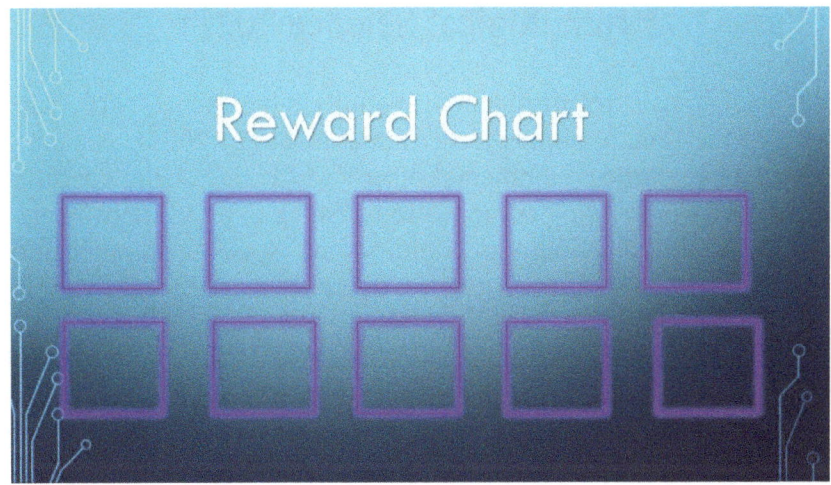

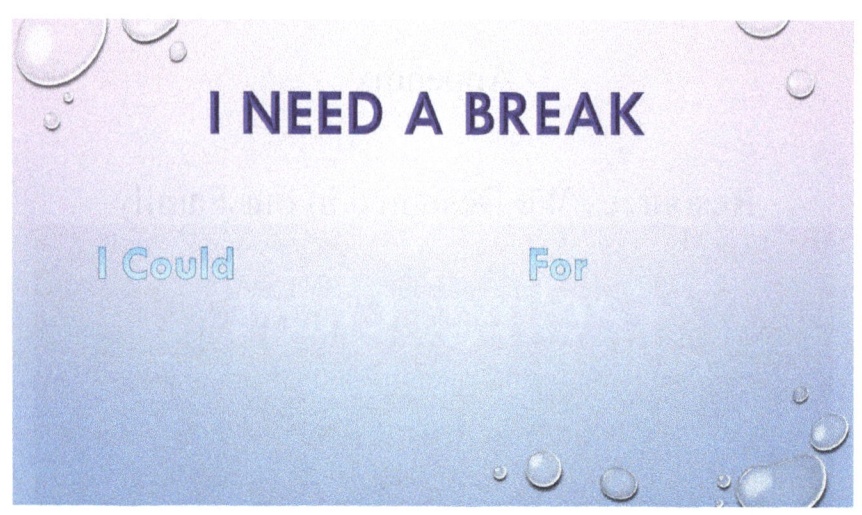

Literature Review on PMDD and Autism (submitted as part of the Graduate Diploma of Psychological Science 2021)

Diagnosis of autism amongst adults is increasing, particularly amongst the female population (Karavidas et al., 2021). Autism is defined as a neurodevelopmental disorder affecting social cognition with sensory processing complications (Stagg et al., (2019). Autism presents with behaviours of rigidity and social communication difficulties potentially impacting on overall quality of life (Moseley et al., 2020).

Autism diagnosis in late adulthood may affect mental health (Moseley et al. 2020a). This potentially leads to social isolation and a higher vulnerability to suicidality (Moseley et al., 2020a & b). Increasing rates of diagnosis among female children and adults may result in comorbidities such as anxiety and depression throughout the lifespan consequently reducing skills in executive functioning (Moseley et al., 2020b).

Menopause occurs between the ages of 40 to 54 years and is characterised by cessation of the menstrual cycle (Barati et al., 2021). Quality of life during the menopausal period has been subject to difficulties in the domains of physical, social and mental health, based on hormonal fluctuations and the state of health prior to menopause (Barati et al., 2021). Given the rigidity, social communication difficulties and sensory complications attributed to a diagnosis of autism, Moseley et al. (2020b) explored the connection between engagement in masking behaviours, defined as covering social impairment and sensory stimulation overload, during the onset of menopause. They predicted a further decline in quality of life and an inability to engage in masking behaviours.

Moseley et al. (2020a)'s initial pilot study of 17 females revealed severe deficits in the areas of health and wellbeing, prompting further studies into the association between masking, menopause and autism. Concurring with this, Karavidas et al. (2021)'s study of seven women revealed similarities between the experience of late diagnosis of autism and menopause. Results indicate an inability to engage in masking behaviours when transitioning through the menopausal period (Moseley et al., 2020a&b). Currently there is very limited research in this area. Furthermore, there has been no research between masking, autism and premenstrual dysphoric disorder, PMDD, a disorder affecting 3-5 percent of females impacting the state of mental health during the regular menstrual cycle (Comasco et al., 2020 & Reid 2017).

References

Arnold. S., Huang., Y, Hwang., Y, Richdale, A., Trollor, J., Lawson, L. (2020). The Single Most Important Thing That Has Happened to Me in My Life": Development of the Impact of Diagnosis Scale - Preliminary Revision, Autism in Adulthood. Volume 2, Number 1, Mary Ann Liebert, Inc. DOI: 10.1089/aut.2019.0059

Azizi, Z., 2015. What is Autism? DOI:10.13140/RG.2.1.5096.1123

Barati, M., Akbari-heidari, H., Samadi-yaghin, E. (2021). The factors associated with the quality of life among postmenopausal women. *BMC Women's Health* 21, 208 https://doi.org/10.1186/s12905-021-01361-x

Braun, V. & Clarke, V., (2006). Using thematic analysis in psychology. Qualitative Research in Psychology *Edward Arnold (Publishers) Ltd*; 3: 77_/101.

Braun, V. & Clarke, V., (2019). Reflecting on reflexive thematic analysis, Qualitative Research in Sport, Exercise and Health, Routledge, Taylor & Francis Group, 11:4, 589-597

Cage, E. & Troxell- Whitman, Z. (2020). Understanding the Relationships Between Autistic Identity, Disclosure, and Camouflaging. *Autism in Adulthood.* Volume 2, Number 4, Mary Ann Liebert, Inc.DOI: 10.1089/aut.2020.0016

Comasco, E., Kopp Kallner, H., Bixo, M., Hirschberg, A., Nyback,S., de Grauw, H., Epperson, N., Sundström-Poromaa, I. (2020). Ulipristal Acetate for Treatment of Premenstrual Dysphoric Disorder: A Proof-of-Concept Randomized Controlled Trial. American Journal of Psychiatry, appi.ajp.2020.2 DOI: 10.1176/appi.ajp.2020.20030286

Dissanayake, C., Richdale, A., Kolivas., N & Pamment, L. (2019). An Exploratory Study of Autism Traits and Parenting Journal of Autism and Developmental Disorders. 50:2593–2606 https://doi.org/10.1007/s10803-019-03984-4

Dudas RB, Lovejoy C, Cassidy S, Allison C, Smith P, Baron-Cohen S (2017) The overlap between autistic spectrum conditions and borderline personality disorder. PLoS ONE 12(9): e0184447. https://doi.org/10.1371/journal.pone.0184447

Hodges., H., Fealko. C, Soares. N., (2019) Autism spectrum disorder: definition, epidemiology, causes, and clinical evaluation. Translational Pediatrics. http://dx.doi.org/10.21037/tp.2019.09.09

Karavidas, M., & de Visser, R. O. (2021). "It's Not Just in My Head, and It's Not Just Irrelevant": Autistic Negotiations of Menopausal Transitions. Journal of autism and developmental disorders, 10.1007/s10803-021-05010-y. Advance online publication. https://doi.org/10.1007/s10803-021-05010-y

McDonald. T. (2020). Autism Identity and the "Lost Generation": Structural Validation of the Autism Spectrum Identity Scale and Comparison of Diagnosed and Self-Diagnosed Adults on the Autism Spectrum. Autism in Adulthood. Volume 2, Number 1, [a] Mary Ann Liebert, Inc. DOI: 10.1089/aut.2019.0069

Miserandino, C. (2003). The Spoon Theory. www.butyoudontlooksick.com

Molloy, C. A., Murray, D. S., Akers, R., Mitchell, T., & Manning-Courtney, P. (2011). Use of the Autism Diagnostic Observation Schedule (ADOS) in a clinical setting. Autism, 15(2), 143–162. https://doi.org/10.1177/1362361310379241

Moseley, R. L., Druce, T., & Turner-Cobb, J. M. (2020a). 'When my autism broke': A qualitative study spotlighting autistic voices on menopause. Autism, 24(6), 1423–1437. https://doi.org/10.1177/1362361319901184Moseley, R. L.,

Druce, T., & Turner-Cobb, J. M. (2020b). Autism research is 'all about the blokes and the kids': Autistic women breaking the silence on menopause. British Journal of Health Psychology (IF3.311), Pub Date : 2020-09-30, DOI: 10.1111/bjhp.12477

Nowell. L.S, Norris. J.M, White. D.E & Moules. N.J. (2017). Thematic Analysis: Striving to Meet the Trustworthiness Criteria. International Journal of Qualitative Methods. Sage Publications. DOI: 10.1177/1609406917733847

Pearson, A., & Rose., K. (2021). A Conceptual Analysis of Autistic Masking: Understanding the Narrative of Stigma and the Illusion of Choice. Autism in Adulthood. Vol 3, No 1, DOI: 10.1089/aut.2020.0043

Pelicano, E. Lawson,W., Hall, G., Mahony,J., Lilley,R., Davis, C., Arnold, S., Trollor, J. & Yudell, M. (2020). Documenting the untold histories of late-diagnosed autistic adults: a qualitative study protocol using oral history methodology. BMJ Open. doi:10.1136/bmjopen-2020-037968

Raymaker, D., Teo, A., Steckler, N., Lentz, B., Scharer, M., Santos, A., Kapp, S., Hunter, M., Joyce, A. & Nicolaidis, C., (2021). "Having All of Your Internal Resources Exhausted Beyond Measure and Being Left with No Clean-Up Crew": Defining Autistic Burnout Autism in Adulthood. Volume 2, Number 2, Mary Ann Liebert, Inc. DOI: 10.1089/aut.2019.0079

Reid RL. (2017), Premenstrual Dysphoric Disorder (Formerly Premenstrual Syndrome) In: Feingold KR, Anawalt B, Boyce A, et al., editors. Endotext [Internet]. South Dartmouth (MA): MDText.com, Inc.; 2000-. Table 1, Diagnostic Criteria for Premenstrual Dysphoric Disorder (PMDD) Available from: https://www.ncbi.nlm.nih.gov/books/NBK279045/table/premenstrual-syndrom.table1diag/

Sedwick, F., Crane, L., Hill, V. & Pellicano, E., (2020). Friends and lovers: the relationships of autistic and neurotypical women. Autism in Adulthood.

Stagg, D. & Belcher. H. (2019). Living with autism without knowing: receiving a diagnosis in later life. Health Psychology and Behavioral Medicine. 7:1, 348-361, DOI:10.1080/21642850.2019.1684920

Tong. A., Sainsbury P, & Craig, J. (2019) Consolidated criteria for reporting qualitative research (COREQ): a 32-item checklist for interviews and focus groups. International Journal for Quality in Health Care vol. 19 no. 6

Lightning Source UK Ltd.
Milton Keynes UK
UKHW022322130622
404374UK00006B/184